DATE DUE

FEB 1 2 2002	

Long-Term Care Decisions

Long-Term Care Decisions

Ethical and Conceptual Dimensions

edited by

Laurence B. McCullough
Center for Ethics, Medicine, and Public Issues
and Huffington Center on Aging

and

Nancy L. Wilson
Huffington Center on Aging

BAYLOR COLLEGE OF MEDICINE
HOUSTON, TEXAS

The Johns Hopkins University Press
Baltimore and London

The Johns Hopkins University Press
2715 North Charles Street
Baltimore, Maryland 21218-4319
The Johns Hopkins Press Ltd., London

Library of Congress Cataloging-in-Publication Data will be found at the end of this book.
A catalog record for this book is available from the British Library.

ISBN 0-8018-4993-4

Contents

Preface

Every now and then in the academic life very special moments occur. One such moment in our lives lasted an entire weekend—April 2–4, 1993 to be precise—when the authors of the chapters in this book gathered in Houston for a working conference on the conceptual and ethical dimensions of long-term care decision making. This conference grew out of our longstanding interest in ethics in long-term care and the work on this subject of the Ethics Research Group of the Baylor College of Medicine Huffington Center on Aging. The goal of the Ethics Research Group has been and continues to be to merge complementary interests and skills—of philosophy, social work, medicine, and public health—in the study of ethics and aging.

Our colleagues prepared and sent their papers in advance of the conference, read them carefully, and gave themselves over to an extraordinary conversation about their papers and the issues they raised. With great pleasure we now lay before the reader the results of this weekend of scholarly work, intellectual exhilaration, superb conversation, and Texas cuisine.

This conference also had its origins in a grant to Baylor College of Medicine's Huffington Center on Aging from the UpJohn Foundation. Our colleagues in the Huffington Center very generously suggested that the funds should be used for a conference on ethics in aging, in support of the then fledgling Ethics Research Group. As we thought about appropriate topics, we realized that there was clearly a movement afoot in the literature on ethics and aging. Recent scholarship had taken an initial move beyond the "four-alarm" issues surrounding death and dying and beyond the attention-grabbing issues of rationing health care resources for the elderly to a topic that involves millions of elders and their families, long-term care decision making. We invited our colleagues to a working conference with the goals of consolidating that movement, building on it, pushing the envelope of both long-term care concepts and practice, and challenging core concepts of bioethics. We believe that our colleagues have more than succeeded in achieving these goals.

We knew that any innovative, trail-blazing investigation of the conceptual and ethical dimensions of long-term care decision making would have to be interdisciplinary. Now, "interdisciplinary" has become something of a shibboleth. We sought to make it a working reality for this conference and the book that we expected to issue from the conference. And so we asked our colleagues to prepare their papers in a genuine interdisciplinary spirit and to devote our time together in the working conference to intense, searching discussion of their papers. The resulting process took on the character of "self-editing," as John Arras put it at one point. As a consequence, the chapters that follow exhibit a high degree of integration. We think that they represent interdisciplinary work in gerontology and in bioethics at its very best. The hard work of our colleagues toward this end made our work as organizers of the conference and editors of this volume truly rewarding work.

The conference and this book would not have come about without the steadfast support and dedicated work of many of our colleagues. We want to acknowledge Robert J. Luchi, Director of the Huffington Center on Aging, and Baruch A. Brody, Director of the Center for Ethics, Medicine, and Public Issues of the Baylor College of Medicine for their commitment to the development of the Ethics Research Group and, in particular, to the working conference that led to this book. The support of the UpJohn Foundation was crucial, and we want especially to thank Leon Rochen of the UpJohn Company and our colleague in the Huffington Center on Aging, Robert E. Roush, whose efforts helped to secure this funding. James R. Smith, also of the Huffington Center, suggested the dedication of the UpJohn funds to a project on ethics in aging when he surely could have claimed them for cell and molecular biology of aging. We esteem him as a scientist and teacher and want to thank him here for his generosity of spirit and collegiality. We also want especially to thank our colleagues in the Ethics Research Group, Thomas A. Teasdale and Jill A. Rhymes, for their collegiality and good humor throughout this and other projects.

We were assisted in the planning process for the conference by four colleagues whose work appears here: John Arras, Nancy Jecker, Rosalie Kane, and Terrie Wetle. Their suggestions and criticisms helped us to sharpen the focus of the working conference and encouraged us to invite our colleagues to challenge orthodoxy and see where doing so would take us: off the accepted conceptual map and into new intellectual territory.

We are especially grateful to current and former administrative staff members of the Huffington Center on Aging for their many hours of unstinting and cheerful work on the numerous, demanding, and sometimes frustrating administrative tasks so essential to a smooth-running conference and the preparation of a book-length manuscript. This project could not have been completed without the very able assistance of Terry Saulsberry. Thank you also to Cynthia Nelson, Karen Mandel, Sue Parker, Nancy Philips, and Patricia White.

The reviewer of the manuscript for the Johns Hopkins University Press gave generously of time and effort to read all of the papers from the conference—now the chapters that follow—to consider them carefully and to comment on them with critical insight and scholarly acumen. The work of the authors of these chapters was much improved by this unstinting collegial effort. We also want to thank our editor at the Press, Wendy Harris, for her support and guidance throughout the process of preparing this book for publication.

As long-term care researchers who recognize the value of family, we thank our spouses, Linda Quintanilla and John Dickinson, and Nancy's children, Philip and Amanda Dickinson, for giving lovingly of their time and support while we undertook our editorial chores.

We would be remiss if we failed to acknowledge two of the great cultural institutions in our city, Felix Restaurant and Goode Company Barbeque, for provisioning us on our intellectual trail ride. Never was the Texas culinary art devoted to higher intellectual and artistic purpose.

The working conference, among many other wonderful things, celebrated the traditions of scholarship and the intellectual life in service to humanity, collegiality, and friendship. We hold the authors of the chapters in this volume in the highest regard and abiding affection. This book really belongs to them.

Contributors

George J. Agich, Ph.D., is Professor of Medical Humanities and Psychiatry and Director of the Medical Ethics Program at Southern Illinois University School of Medicine, Springfield, Illinois, and Director of the Ethics Consultation Service at Memorial Medical Center. He is the author of *Autonomy and Long-Term Care* (1993), editor of *Responsibility in Health Care* (1982), and coeditor of *The Price of Health* (1986). His recent work has focused on the problems of autonomy, competence, and consent among elders. He is also Vice-President of the Association for the Advancement of Philosophy and Psychiatry.

John D. Arras, Ph.D., is Associate Professor in the Division of Bioethics and Health Policy of the Department of Epidemiology and Social Medicine of the Montefiore Medical Center and Albert Einstein College of Medicine, Bronx, New York. He is co-editor of *Ethical Issues in Modern Medicine*, now in its fourth edition (1995), and editor of *Bringing the Hospital Home: Ethical and Social Implications of High-Tech Home Care* (1995). Current research interests include methodological issues in practical ethics, reproductive ethics, and ethical issues in long-term care.

Sarah Vaughan Brakman, Ph.D., is Assistant Professor of Philosophy at Villanova University, Philadelphia, Pennsylvania. She has presented and published papers in the area of health policy in the United States and Europe. Her research interests include ethical issues in medicine and science dealing with the aged, children, mental illness, and health policy. She has been a member of institutional animal care and use committees and is presently a member of the Ethics Committee at Graduate Hospital of Philadelphia.

Thomas R. Cole, Ph.D., is Professor and Graduate Program Director at the Institute for the Medical Humanities, University of Texas Medical Branch, Galveston, Texas. He is author of *The Journey of Life: A Cultural History of Aging* (1992) and senior editor of *What Does*

It Mean to Grow Old: Reflections of the Humanities and Aging;
Voice and Vision: Toward a Critical Gerontology (1993), and *Oxford Book of Aging* (1995).

Bart J. Collopy, Ph.D., is Associate for Ethical Studies at the Third Age Gerontology Center and Associate Professor in the Humanities Division, Fordham University, Bronx, New York. He has served on a number of ethics committees on long-term care and has written extensively on ethical issues in both institutional and community-based care for the elderly.

Martha Holstein, M.A., is currently a doctoral student at the Institute for the Medical Humanities, University of Texas Medical Branch, Galveston, Texas. She has served as Associate Director of the American Society on Aging and Western Coordinator of the Hastings Center. She has coedited (with Paul Homer) a book on health care rationing, *A Good Old Age? The Paradox of Setting Limits* (1990), and has authored a number of articles and book chapters on aging-related topics.

Nancy S. Jecker, Ph.D., is Associate Professor, Department of Medical History and Ethics, University of Washington School of Medicine and Adjunct Associate Professor in the School of Law and Department of Philosophy, University of Washington, Seattle, Washington. She is editor of *Aging and Ethics: Philosophical Problems in Gerontology* (1991) and has written 46 articles and 23 book chapters on topics such as ethics and aging, ethics and the family, and justice in the allocation of health care resources. She recently completed a book with Lawrence J. Schneiderman, *Wrong Medicine: The Pursuit of Futile Treatments* (1995).

Rosalie A. Kane, D.S.W., is Professor of Public Health at the University of Minnesota, where she is also on the faculty of the Center for Biomedical Ethics and the School of Social Work. She directs the University of Minnesota's Long-Term Care Resource Center, one of four such Centers funded by the Administration on Aging in 1993. Her research emphases center around health, personal care, and social services for the elderly and other dependent groups, including quality of care, assessment, care management, home care, nursing home care, and, more recently, the study of values and ethics. Between 1988 and 1992 she was Editor-in-Chief of *The Gerontologist.* With Robert Kane she has coauthored five books: *Long-Term Care: Prin-*

ciples, Programs and Policies (1987), *A Will and a Way: What the United States Can Learn from Canada about Caring for the Elderly* (1985), *Values and Long-Term Care* (1982), *Assessing the Elderly: A Practical Guide to Measurement* (1981), and *Long-Term Care in Six Countries: Implications for the United States* (1976). With Arthur Caplan she is coeditor of *Everyday Ethics: Resolving Dilemmas in Nursing Home Life* (1990) and *Ethical Conflicts in the Management of Home Care: The Case Manager's Dilemma* (1993).

Laurence B. McCullough, Ph.D., is Professor of Medicine, Community Medicine, and Medical Ethics in the Center for Ethics, Medicine, and Public Issues and Faculty Associate in the Huffington Center on Aging, Baylor College of Medicine in Houston, Texas. He is an Adjunct Research Fellow in the Institute of Religion of the Texas Medical Center and a former President of the Society for Health and Human Values (1987 to 1988). He is coauthor (with Frank A. Chervenak, M.D.) of *Ethics in Obstetrics and Gynecology* (1994) and coauthor or coeditor of six other books, including (with Tom L. Beauchamp) *Medical Ethics: The Moral Responsibilities of Physicians* (1984), which has been translated into Spanish (1987) and Japanese (1992).

Jill A. Rhymes, M.D., is a geriatrician trained at Mt. Sinai Medical Center in New York City in geriatrics. She is Director of the Geriatric Evaluation and Management Unit and the Geriatrics Consult Service at the Houston Veterans Affairs Medical Center and is an Assistant Professor of Medicine at Baylor College of Medicine. She is also Faculty Associate of Baylor's Huffington Center on Aging. She has written on hospice care in America and pain management for dying patients. Her current research interests include values in long-term care decision making and the professional's role in long-term care decision making.

Thomas A. Teasdale, M.P.H., is Biostatistician for Geriatrics and Extended Care Service of the Houston Veterans Affairs Medical Center, Faculty Associate in the Huffington Center on Aging of Baylor College of Medicine, and Research Instructor in the Department of Medicine, Baylor College of Medicine, Houston, Texas. He expects to be awarded the Dr.P.H. degree from the University of Texas by the time that this work appears in print. His doctoral research involved a concentration in aging studies and investigation of the capacity of cognitively impaired elders to prepare advance directives. He has published and made presentations at professional meetings in the fields of geriatrics and gerontology for more than ten years.

Terrie Wetle, Ph.D., was the Director for the Braceland Center for Mental Health and Aging at the Institute of Living in Hartford, Connecticut. She is also Associate Professor of Community Medicine and Medical Health and Director of the Research Curriculum for the Travelers Center on Aging in the School of Medicine at the University of Connecticut in Farmington, Connecticut. She has held positions previously at Harvard Medical School, Yale University, Portland State University, and the federal government. Dr. Wetle has served with distinction on a number of private boards and state and federal commissions on Alzheimer's disease and long-term care. Her research interests include social gerontology, the organization and financing of health care, and ethical issues in geriatric care. She has more than eighty scientific publications and serves on the editorial boards of several scholarly journals. She presently is Deputy Director of the National Institute on Aging.

Nancy L. Wilson, M.A., is Instructor of Geriatric Medicine and Assistant Director for Program Development of the Huffington Center on Aging, Baylor College of Medicine in Houston, Texas. She is also Clinical Coordinator for the Texas Consortium of Geriatric Education Centers and Lecturer in Gerontological Social Work at the University of Houston. As a practitioner for several years, she directed community care programs for elders and family, including serving as Director of the Houston site of the National Long-Term Care Channeling Demonstration. She has written a number of articles and chapters and was an editor of *Aging 2000: Our Healthcare Destiny —Psychosocial and Policy Issues* (1985).

Long-Term Care Decisions

Rethinking the Conceptual and Ethical Dimensions of Long-Term Care Decision Making

Laurence B. McCullough and Nancy L. Wilson

This book is about the conceptual and ethical dimensions of long-term care decision making. Its authors take a decidedly "downwards-up" approach (Brody, 1990), beginning with the history and policy constraints of long-term care decisions, the experience of case managers and other long-term care professionals, and the experiences of elders and their families—not with abstract philosophical theories already assumed to be adequate to the task. The authors thus mount a challenge to methodologies in bioethics that are separated from history, policy, and practice. In the process, they challenge received assumptions about such key concepts as autonomy, safety, independence, interpersonal relations based on kinship ties, and conflicts of interest. Thus, this book is also about more than long-term care decision making.

Long-term care has been described as "a set of health, personal care and social services delivered over a sustained period of time to persons who have lost or never acquired some degree of functional capacity" (Kane and Kane, 1987, p. 4). This book targets long-term care decision making by elders, family members, and professionals. Thus, it is about long-term care decision making at what might usefully be termed the "micro" level of individuals, of everyday life. Obviously, the microlevel of decision making about long-term care is affected by "macrolevel" considerations of public policy and of institutional practice and policy.

Long-term care decision making involves millions of elders, family members, and professionals every year in the United States (and other countries). These decisions concern at the least (*a*) where an elder with long-term care needs should live—for example, continue to live in his or her home or apartment or move to congregate housing or even a nursing home; (*b*) what sort of care the elder needs and ought therefore to have—for example, stimulation that a day care program might provide or nutrition from a Meals-on-Wheels program; and (*c*) who ought to provide either the location of long-term care or long-term care services.

For example, the decision by a frail elder who has experienced a fall at home followed by hospitalization to move in with her adult daughter and her family may follow a period of time in the hospital and in a nursing home utilized by the hospital as a step-down, transitional setting. The elder and her family confront a host of quotidian decisions about such matters as finances, where pets will go, family work schedules, living space, and meal contents and schedules. The decision-making process can be further complicated by the elder's actual or perceived diminished ability—or even inability—to make decisions, as a result of physical or mental changes that have been occurring. The elder may thus in some cases not be able to participate meaningfully in the decision-making process. Decision makers also grapple with conflicting interests, uneven distribution of caregiving burdens, especially by gender, an uncertain sense of spousal and filial obligations and their limits, lack of clarity about roles and power, and emotional conflicts between and within decision makers. The people involved in the process can change over time. Decision makers may also hold sharply different views of the elder's problems and needs and of their own capacities to meet those needs.

Long-term care decision making is thus an enormously, though not hopelessly, complex process, because it involves a series of medical, social, and personal decisions, made incrementally over time by multiple decision makers, rather than a single, well-defined, time-bound decision made, as in acute care, by the dyad of physician and patient. The conceptual and ethical dimensions of microlevel long-term care decision making have begun to attract the attention and investigation of scholars in gerontology, geriatrics, and bioethics. The purpose of this book is, in a highly integrated interdisciplinary effort, to identify the key conceptual and ethical dimensions of long-term care decision making, their implications for practice, and a preventive ethics approach to managing the conceptual and ethical dimensions of long-term care decision making.

Part of our purpose in bringing this volume into print is to complement recent work on macrolevel long-term care decision making with a sustained look at microlevel long-term care decision making by elders, their families, and professionals (Dunkle and Wykle, 1988; Eisdorfer, Kessler, and Specter, 1989; Harrington et al., 1985; Kane and Kane, 1982; Kane and Kane, 1987; Leutz et al., 1992). A more important purpose is to make a contribution that fills a gap in the literature on ethics and aging.

There is, to be sure, a growing literature on ethics and aging, making significant contributions to the bioethics as well as gerontologic and geriatric literature. Until very recently—and to some extent still as we write—the literature of ethics and aging is dominated by end-of-life decision making regarding such matters as futile medical management, refusal of critical care interventions through such legal instruments as the living will and durable power of attorney, and physician-assisted suicide.

Important correctives to this imbalance in the ethics and aging literature have appeared in the past five years. These include first-rate scholarly collections on everyday ethical issues in nursing home care (Kane and Caplan, 1990), ethical issues in home care (Kane and Caplan, 1993), ethical concerns in caring for geriatric patients with dementing diseases and disorders (Binstock, Post, and Whitehouse, 1992), family caregiving (Cicirelli, 1992), as well as general ethical issues in aging (Jecker, 1991). In addition, there have recently appeared careful, philosophical studies of key concepts in ethics and aging (Moody, 1992) and in long-term care decision making (Agich, 1993; Lidz, Fischer, and Arnold, 1993). These were preceded by Bart Collopy's pioneering work (1986), which was supported by an initiative on ethics and aging undertaken a decade ago by the Retirement Research Foundation (Hofland, 1988; Hofland, 1990)—the effect of that initiative was far-reaching, influencing much of the work that appears in this volume—and work in ethical issues in chronic illness (Jennings, Callahan, and Caplan, 1988).

This growing body of literature has created the need for an explicitly interdisciplinary examination of the several conceptual and ethical dimensions of long-term care decision making. To that end the ten chapters that follow (*a*) ground the analyses of subsequent chapters in a well-informed policy, political, and historical context; (*b*) further ground the explorations that follow in empirical accounts of the ethical issues confronted by professionals working with elders and their families on the long-term care decision making process; (*c*) examine in the next two chapters the basic concepts of autonomy, independence, and safety; (*d*) explore in three chapters the tangled web of spousal and filial obligations, the legitimate interests of family members, and the obligations of elders; and (*e*) in all chapters mount a series of challenges to accepted concepts in long-term care practice and in bioethics.

These ten chapters provide the basis for a translation of the conceptual and ethical dimensions of long-term care decision making into their practice implications. These implications take the form of an ethically justified preventive ethics strategy for managing the conceptual and ethical dimensions of long-term care decision making.

A Precis of the Book
Contextual Considerations

Martha Holstein and Thomas Cole begin with a historical examination and analysis of the hidden values and social forces that have shaped long-term care services, a topic usually missing from discussions of ethics in long-term care. These values and forces provide the larger context in which long-term care decision making occurs. Changing attitudes toward old age and dependency during old age, the constancy of family (spousal and filial) obligations and family support, and the reinforcement and exploitation by American society and government of family obligations are central themes. Other historical factors include: the notion of the elder's responsibility to his or her own community; the persistence of "indoor" or institutional versus "outdoor" or community-based responses to long-term care problems; the stigma of the nursing home; compassionate response to long-term care problems in conflict with the disvalue of encouraging dependence; and the persistent link between publicly supported long-term care and poverty. These and other factors discussed by Holstein and Cole provide the historical context for the conceptual and ethical issues discussed in subsequent chapters. Indeed, the history of long-term care in the United States leads directly to long-term care as a public issue and long-term care decision making as ethically problematic.

Nancy Wilson provides an overview of long-term care in the United States, focusing on the elderly client population needing assistance and the pivotal role of family members, especially women, in meeting those needs. The information she presents highlights the view of long-term care as a "normal risk of growing old" and the importance of addressing the conceptual and ethical dimensions of decisions that confront growing numbers of older people and family members. In an examination of current approaches to the organization and financing of long-term care

Wilson notes the "mismatch" between the preferences of older people for continued community residence and public financing of services that has primarily funded institutional services and linked this support to welfare programs. Although some states have developed an expanded array of home- and community-based services, the current expectation of public policy is that elderly individuals and their families must bear the largest share of the physical and economic burdens of chronic illness and functional limitations.

Practice Considerations

Terrie Wetle addresses the ethical issues faced by case managers, who play an increasingly powerful role in long-term care decision making. She notes that, right from the start, the elder-case manager relationship is marked by factors that can adversely affect the elder's autonomy: the "heterogeneity of preferences" among elders about their own participation in decision making, the involvement of family in decision making, and policy and institutional constraints on the nature and extent of the services that might be arranged for the elder to receive. The autonomy of the elder is at risk for being undermined in subtle ways. The case manager must be attentive to this, especially because the case manager, as Wetle repeatedly emphasizes, wields growing power that is shaped as much by concerns of safety and benefit as by respect for the elder's autonomy. Wetle's concerns and cautions are, we believe, generalizable to other professionals' involvement in long-term care decision making, especially the professional's power.

Wetle's chapter reflects a central theme of this volume, namely, that the ethics of long-term care decision making are mainly to be understood in process terms. Her discussion of that process foreshadows the theme in later chapters of the professional's role in allocating the power and degrees of that power to participate in decision making among all of the decision makers, including the case manager. Thus, "Who among family members should be involved?", "How should a case manager respond to an agency's policies regarding financially attractive clients?", and "How should a professional respond to institutional constraints on respect for the client's or patient's autonomy?" become central questions of the morality of the power of professionals in the long-term care decision–making process. In confronting such issues the health care professional involved in long-term care decision making must also confront multiple agency. Wetle portrays potential conflicts that must be managed in an ethically justified fashion by the professional to protect the professionals, as well as the elder, family members, and institutions, from moral incoherence. Absent such strategies, the professional's exercise of power— for or against elders, their families, and agencies—is at inherent risk of abuse. Wetle identifies a key element of a preventive ethics strategy for this problem, namely for the professional to disclose multiple agency and its contradictions as part of the informed consent process for the case manager's involvement in the decision-making process.

Rosalie Kane examines the complexity and elusiveness of long-term care decisions and identifies a myriad of influences on these decisions, particularly including the power of the professional to frame issues and alternatives about both large and small decisions. Through the application of research on decision making to long-term care decisions, a distinctive contribution of this chapter, she becomes the first of several authors in this volume to underscore features of long-term care decision making that are problematic, such as the presence of time pressures and the absence of complete information about alternatives, especially about the benefits *and* risks of each. Kane explores whether it is feasible and desirable for professionals involved in long-term care decision making to undertake systematic efforts to learn the values of their elders and family members and to incorporate such information into the development and delivery of care plans. Drawing on the early lessons of a demonstration project involving attention to values by case managers, Kane identifies the potential for routine inquiry about the values of elders and family members as a way to redress the imbalance of power among elders, family members, and professionals involved in long-term care decision making.

Rethinking Basic Concepts

The conceptual dimensions of long-term care decision making include some of the well-known concepts of long-term care and of biomedical ethics or bioethics, but those concepts need to be rethought, according to virtually every chapter that follows Kane's. Concepts such as autonomy, safety, and independence are drawn too starkly and too abstractly in the bioethics literature to be adequate to the complex and shifting realities of long-term care decision making. As a consequence, a systematic move toward moral ambiguity and its management are essential to understanding the conceptual dimensions of long-term care decision making.

George Agich introduces useful and powerful distinctions that challenge accepted views in bioethics. Nodal decision making is about paradigm events, the clear-cut world of acute care and the idealized, abstract concept of autonomy as self-determination that dominates the bioethics literature. Interstitial decision making is about typical events, the events of everyday life, including many—if not most—long-term care events. They are nothing special and hence not necessarily perceived to be problematic in the way that total hip replacement becomes something special and is often considered problematic. The ideal, abstract concept of autonomy is not adequate to interstitial decision making. Instead, autonomy involves a more nuanced, complicated set of personal characteristics and activities, including "habit and disposition," "enactments," character, "developed patterns" of behavior, an "engaged and preoccupied" life, identification with things, people, and activity, and "adaptive effort."

On such a conceptual account respect for autonomy is not something abstract, as it is in self-determination exercised in the refusal of life-saving treatment (the paradigm of autonomy in the bioethics literature). Instead, respect for autonomy is at once more concrete and more supple: to "foster the effort of elders to reorient themselves by active cooperation in the elders' effort to remake their world." The routine and the ordinary are the grist for autonomy in long-term care, not the dramatic, "four-alarm" issues of intensive care units and emergency departments. In the latter settings, perhaps, patients are strangers. In long-term care, intimacy is a basic ethical category, and respect for autonomy takes this into account by emphasizing actual autonomy in the everyday provision and experience of long-term care.

Bart Collopy deftly argues that independence and safety are only at first glance polar opposites, mounting a challenge to a common assumption in long-term care. Up close, they should be understood as marking the ends of a continuum of effort on the part of elders to give as much meaning and as much coherence to their lives as possible as they face the increasing probability of dependence that marks long-term care problems. Indeed, failing to understand that independence and safety are conceptually and practically related, rather than opposites, could lead to a misunderstanding of long-term care decisions as necessarily involving a forced choice between independence and safety. Rather, Collopy argues, the task is to forge new, richer concepts of independence and safety. These, in turn, serve as the basis of long term care decision making that aims to respect and carry forward as much of the elder's world of meaning as possible, despite powerful institutional and policy constraints that mitigate against doing so. The narrowness of an either/or dichotomy between independence and safety should be replaced by the "conceptual largesse" that sees them, instead, as arrayed in a continuum within which fragile trade-offs are negotiated case by case.

Family Roles and Responsibilities

Nancy Jecker explores the related topic of what married couples owe each other in old age, a crucial ethical dimension of long-term care decision making, given the large role that spouses, female spouses especially, play as informal caregivers. This has been almost completely neglected in the literature. Marriage is understood to be a vital relationship, a dance of two, of love, and of commitment to a particular person. This is obviously a morally demanding social institution, but, again, not one of duty. Caregiving involves not just meeting one's spouse's needs but also making sense of the marriage relationship in the context of its history and in response to changes that occasion long-term care responses. Part of that making sense is taking account of "justified self-concern" because this is an ethically essential component of caregiving generally. In particular, caregiving need not be seen as a career, especially an obligatory career with no limits and especially for female spouses (and female caregivers generally). Caregiving without reprieve threatens and does not sustain marriage, because such caregiving unjustifiably threatens legitimate self-interest and self-respect of the caregiver, turning the obligation of caregiving into the tyrannous vice of endless self-sacrifice. The implicit expectation of public policy that spousal caregiving should become an all-consuming career is thus called sharply into question. Indeed, a central task of long-term care decision making is to negotiate limits on spousal obligations to provide long-term care, especially those of the female spouse.

Sarah Vaughan Brakman mounts a formidable challenge to the notion that reciprocity should be the basis of filial obligations, the obligations that adult children owe to their parents. Instead, gratitude should be understood to ground those obligations. The core of gratitude is the cultivation of virtue, the virtue of the grateful recipient—grateful that, when vulnerable and in need, one was protected and nurtured (at least to some nominal, if not generous degree, by one's parents). One is thus always bound to one's parents, in the regard with which one should hold them. But one is not therefore necessarily bound by limitless obligations to meet parental needs, as an adult child might be under reciprocity to a parent who had sacrificed a great deal in rearing his or her children. No hard and fast line, no clear-cut criteria define those limits. Given the variability in which the magnitude of gratitude (i.e., what is owed) is understood, those limits must be negotiated on a case-by-case basis in long-term care decision making. Brakman identifies some important ethical implications of gratitude for this process, including recognition of competing obligations of an adult child to others, the adult child's own projects and goals, and the more equal distribution across genders of caregiving burdens.

Brakman's and Jecker's analyses converge in the idea that there are legitimate limits that adult children and spouses, especially female adult children and spouses, can and should place on their family obligations. These should not be understood as *conflicts* of interest but rather as the assertion of legitimate interests. John Arras undertakes to map the complex and shifting terrain of conflict of interest in long-term care decision making, in which "we reach the outer boundary of the exclusively patient-centered moral framework of acute care medicine, a boundary where interesting and important questions remain unanswered." Indeed, that moral framework is challenged and found wanting. When family members are themselves direct caregivers, Arras suggests, their conflicts of interest should not be understood—as it seems to be in the acute care, hospital setting—to be in and of themselves disabling of their moral authority to participate in decision making. Instead, the task is that of an "ethic of accommodation": to discern whether a decision by family members that runs counter to the patient's preferences should be understood as a situation in which family members' interests "count for something *in their own right*" and therefore might in some cases justifiably override the interests of the elder with long-term care needs. This, too, becomes a central element of the preventive ethics approach to long-term care decision making that is described in the final chapter.

Preventive Ethics in Long-Term Care Decision Making

In the closing chapter, with our colleagues in the Ethics Research Group of the Baylor College of Medicine Huffington Center on Aging, we challenge the reactive approach to ethical conflicts that presently dominates the bioethics and therefore ethics and aging literature. Instead, we propose a preventive ethics approach to long-term care decision making. The authors base this approach on a carefully drawn distinction of long-term care from acute care and the identification of the practice implications of the previous nine chapters. They also go on to mount a challenge to the core of bioethics, acute, high-tech medicine, from its periphery, long-term care.

Six Common Themes

At least six themes are common to the chapters that follow, joining them into a coherent, clinically applicable whole.

1. Long-term care decision making is a complex, fuzzy process that involves shifting family participants with varying levels of ability and senses of obligation to meet the elder's care needs and various professionals in roles of multiple agency, all working under institutional and policy constraints.

2. The conceptual and ethical dimensions of this process are not well understood, especially if we rely on the conceptual tools of bioethics, which were developed mainly in response to ethical problems in acute care with its singularly patient-centered focus.

3. Any adequate attempt to understand the conceptual and ethical dimensions of long-term care decision making therefore requires that thoroughgoing challenges be mounted to conceptual analyses and ethical frameworks that presently dominate the bioethics literature and therefore the ethics and aging literature.

4. As a consequence, fresh approaches must be developed for the analysis of the conceptual and ethical dimensions of long-term care decision making and therefore of their implications for practice, a goal that is pursued with vigor in the chapters that follow.

5. These fresh philosophical and ethical analyses and arguments about long-term care decision making must be well grounded in empirical studies and in the policy and historical contexts that powerfully shape macrolevel long-term care decision making and, through institutional policies and practices, also powerfully and subtly shape microlevel long-term care decision making.

6. The conceptual and ethical dimensions of long-term care decision making that must be addressed include identifying the appropriate exercise of professional power; addressing historically rooted policy and institutional constraints; rethinking such basic concepts as autonomy and safety and independence; rethinking family roles and responsibilities; and orienting the ethics of long-term care decision making toward a

preventive ethics approach, rooted in the complex moral life of elders, their families, and professionals.

Conclusion

Elders, family members, and professionals engaged in long-term care decision making must recognize and, ideally, grapple with its conceptual and ethical dimensions, because these are built-in, inescapable dimensions of that decision making process. Failure to address these dimensions of long-term care decision making puts that process at risk either for decisions that are poorly made or even imposed on the elder or family or for unnecessary moral turbulence and the intrapsychic and interpersonal stress that inevitably accompanies such upheaval. Simply imposing decisions on others shows profound disrespect for them. Morally turbulent decision-making processes can overwhelm the people involved in them, elders with long-term care needs especially. The following chapters provide the reader with carefully examined and well-argued intellectual and clinical tools to prevent participants in long-term care decision making from simply making decisions or from being overwhelmed by the decision-making process and to direct that process toward the enhancement of the moral lives of all who participate in it. These chapters chart a new course for the ethics of long-term care decision making, and as a consequence, for bioethics generally.

Examining the conceptual and ethical dimensions of long-term care decision making illuminates fundamental questions about how society will respond to the certainty of chronic illness in an aging society whose traditional caregivers, women, are performing other economic and social roles. The cases presented in the chapters that follow remind us that older people are more than the sum of their dependencies; they have their own life histories and goals that may not fit easily into professional and institutional care plans, particularly in a society that endorses institutional care for individuals whose needs outlive or outlast their resources or the resources of their families. The conceptual and ethical dimensions of long-term care decision making that are explored in this book challenge professionals, administrators, and policy makers alike to rethink current approaches to long-term care.

REFERENCES

Agich, G.J. (1993). *Autonomy and Long-Term Care*. New York: Oxford University Press.

Binstock, R.H., Post, S.G., and Whitehouse, P.J. (eds.). (1992). *Dementia and Aging: Ethics, Values, and Policy Choices.* Baltimore: Johns Hopkins University Press.

Brody, B.A. (1990). The quality of scholarship in bioethics. *Journal of Medicine and Philosophy, 15:* 161–178.

Cicirelli, V.G. (1992). *Family Caregiving: Autonomous and Paternalistic Decision Making.* Beverly Hills, Calif.: Sage Publications.

Collopy, B.J. (1986). *The Conceptually Problematic Status of Autonomy: A Report Prepared for the Retirement Research Foundation.*

Dunkle, R.E., and Wykle, M.L. (eds.). (1988). *Decision Making in Long-Term Care: Factors in Planning.* New York: Springer Publishing Co.

Eisdorfer, C., Kessler, P.A., and Specter, A.N. (eds.). (1989). *Caring for the Elderly: Reshaping Public Policy.* Baltimore: Johns Hopkins University Press.

Harrington, C., Newcomer, R.J., Estes, C.L., and Associates. (1985). *Long Term Care of the Elderly.* Beverly Hills, Calif.: Sage Publications.

Hofland, B.F. (1988). Autonomy and long-term care: Background issues and a programmatic response. *Gerontologist, 28:* 3–9.

Hofland, B.F. (ed.). (1990). Autonomy and long-term care practice. *Generations, 14*(Supplement).

Jecker, N.S. (ed.). (1991). *Aging and Ethics.* Clifton, N.J.: Humana Press.

Jennings, B, Callahan, D., and Caplan, A. (1988). Ethical challenges of chronic illness. *Hastings Center Report, 2*(Special Supplement): 1–16.

Kane, R.A., and Caplan, A.L. (eds.). (1990). *Ethical Issues in the Everyday Life of Nursing Home Residents.* New York: Springer Publishing Co.

Kane, R.A., and Caplan, A. L. (eds.). (1993). *Ethical Conflicts in the Management of Home Care: The Case Manager's Dilemma.* New York: Springer Publishing Co.

Kane, R.A. and Kane, R.L. (1982). *Values and Long-Term Care.* Lexington, Mass.: Lexington Books.

Kane, R.A., and Kane, R.L. (1987). *Long-Term Care: Principles, Programs, and Policies.* New York: Springer Publishing Co.

Leutz, W. N., Capitman, J. A., MacAdam, M., and Abrahams, R. (1992). *Care for Frail Elders: Developing Community Solutions.* Westport, Conn.: Auburn House.

Lidz, C.W., Fischer, L., and Arnold, R.M. (1993). *The Erosion of Autonomy in Long-Term Care.* New York: Oxford University Press.

Moody, H.R. (1992). *Ethics and Aging.* Baltimore: Johns Hopkins University Press.

I CONTEXTUAL CONSIDERATIONS

CHAPTER TWO

Long-Term Care: A Historical Reflection

Martha Holstein and Thomas R. Cole

In the late twentieth century long-term care has a commonly understood meaning. It signifies a complex array of institutional and community-based services designed for individuals with physical or mental impairments. Where once, with rare exceptions, women presided over illness and dying at home in the company of other women, today they render that care in relative isolation. Instead of having the communal support of other women, caregivers in the home and in the institution provide care within the formal framework of professional assessment and care planning. The infusion of public funds bespeaks eligibility criteria and accountability.

The gradual transition to modern long-term care occurred in a complex historical context that includes the rise of the welfare state. Although old-age dependence is as ancient as human society, America's public response to such dependence since the eighteenth century reflects specific social relationships and beliefs concerning medicine, old age, indigence, and the relationship of the public and private spheres. Separately and together, these ideologies and the policies they shaped helped structure the conditions in which modern bioethics operates.[1] As such, historical reflection can reveal how largely hidden values and social forces have shaped and limited—and still shape and limit—long-term care choices. Such reflection also reveals pragmatic economic concerns and demographic realities. Our troubles and triumphs have deep roots (Dowling, 1982).

In this chapter, we will sketch the "dominant story" about long-term care, that is, the story of largely middle-class attempts to provide public and voluntary assistance to the poor, the disabled, and the elderly.

Told largely from the perspective of the professional caregiver, this story leads directly to the dilemmas and problems we encounter today in caring for vulnerable and sick older people.

We must emphasize, however, that this dominant story is not *the* history of long-term care. Historians during the last twenty years have acknowledged the impossibility of writing any metanarrative capable of unifying historical experiences from a perspective outside time and society. There are only histories, mostly unwritten, that can be refracted through the prisms of gender, race, class, age, ethnicity, and geographical region, among other variables. Some day many histories of long-term care may be written from "various viewpoints, with many voices, emplotted diversely according to many principles of synthesis" (Berkhofer, 1989, p. 197). Now we have primarily the dominant story to tell, although our essay integrates some material from postbellum African-American communities and highlights the distinct gender assumptions that hid so much of traditional caregiving from public view. Though this story opens in the seventeenth century, its major focus is the nineteenth, a century that changed the complexion, class structure, and culture of America. As such, this story both reflects and reinforces America's historical pattern of racial and ethnic discrimination and class distinctions, a pattern whose ethical consequences remain largely unaddressed.

Our primary story focuses on indigence and infirmity, categories of need that were, for most of our history, age-irrelevant but filled with moralistic judgments of worthiness and unworthiness. We begin with early American "outdoor" relief,[2] an essentially local, flexible, and relatively informal effort to take care of established community residents in their own homes or the homes of others. Beginning in the 1820s, "outdoor" relief, though never abandoned, gave way to "indoor" relief, whose centerpiece was the almshouse. Designed to house the poor and ill of all ages, the almshouse, by the end of the nineteenth century, became a warehouse for the old.

After 1935, long-term care began to assume an increasingly familiar shape. The stepchild of the new ideology of curative medicine, it emerged from the ruins of the much maligned poorhouse. From the beginning, it was governed by a rising professional class who increasingly viewed old age as a medical problem requiring expert attention. This particular combination of factors, which we shall address in greater detail below, has shaped the contemporary ethical problems addressed by this volume. Long-term care has become an important public issue, politically and ethically problematic. Such practical concerns as its limits, its escalating costs, its institutional bias, and its effect on old people and caregiving family members, predominantly women, mingle with equally difficult philosophical and existential questions.

A primary assumption that runs through this history is that families, a euphemism for wives and daughters, would take primary responsibility for their disabled or impoverished elders. This trend has continued. In the last decade of the twentieth century, most people continue to grow old in private homes and neighborhoods, near family and friends. Spousal and filial responsibility, whether offered grudgingly or lovingly, whether expected by law or assumed by choice, has perhaps been one of the most consistent, and until recently most ignored, themes in American history. After 1820, following the general retreat from "outdoor" relief, family caregiving occurred outside the public response to dependency. There it remained, beyond the scope of nineteenth- and early twentieth-century reform movements, until it was rediscovered in the second third of the twentieth century (Benjamin, 1993). Yet even today, the gender and class characteristics of family caregiving are often obscured by the neutral use of "family" and by limited attention to how income affects a family's ability to fulfill its caregiving tasks. These features of long-term care raise questions about gender justice within the family (Okin, 1989), which Nancy Jecker discusses in Chapter 8, as well as larger themes of social justice.

In this chapter we divide the history of long-term care into four roughly defined periods. In the colonial and early republican eras, relief was local, small-scale, noninstitutional, and strongly influenced by Calvinistic beliefs. Older people were generally deemed worthy no matter the life they had formerly led. From 1820 to 1865, relief traveled indoors, that is, to institutions. At once optimistic, zealous, self-righteous, and punitive, reformers adopted policies designed, they believed, to ameliorate pauperism and intemperance. Attitudes toward the aged and views about their worthiness became more complicated in this period. The third period, 1865 to 1935, was far darker. Conditions deteriorated while the almshouse population grayed; profoundly pessimistic beliefs about old age arose. In the more familiar period from 1935 to the present, modern long-term care was born. Emerging from the depression and the birth of the modern nursing home industry, long-term care bore its scarred history into a troubled present.

Colonial and Early Republican America: To the 1820s

Early American families provided virtually all care for poor and infirm elders. Supported by both culture and law, public officials held individuals or members of families accountable. The colonists modeled their system of "outdoor" relief on the familiar English Poor Law of 1601, which held government responsible for giving public relief to those who could not support themselves or obtain support from relatives, friends, or private philanthropy (Quadagno, 1986). Although such relief was rarely munificent, it was generally flexible and dispensed without long investigations, dislocation, or discomfort (Kutzik, 1979). Relief sometimes involved finding work for an ailing man; at other times it meant providing food and lodging when someone's deteriorating health made employment impossible (Quadagno, 1986). Instead of cash, the community might present a family with a milk cow or a piece of land to tide them over (McClure, 1968). In their turn, recipients of poor relief, including the old, were often expected to sew or knit or undertake other modest tasks in keeping with their reduced physical state. Communal values supported *both* rights and responsibilities of the recipients.

Poor old people, whether infirm or able-bodied, were not singled out for categorical assistance. An accepting attitude toward most poor people, especially the aged, the widowed, and the infirm who were also established community residents, made need-based assistance nonstigmatizing and not overwhelmingly niggardly. At the same time, there was no need to distinguish between those who needed help because they were poor and those whose need arose from illness. The limited efficacy of curative medicine made the few existing hospitals little more than another form of poor relief (Rosenberg, 1987).

Communities thus adopted a few relatively simple approaches to meet the needs of older residents. Sometimes such help meant giving aid to very poor families so they could care for their elder relatives. If an elder had no family, he or she might be boarded with a neighbor or neighbors, sometimes in rotation, or the community might ask someone to move in with the older person. And, in an early version of home care, the old and infirm were sometimes assisted in their own homes (Butners, 1980).

For strangers and the able-bodied, however, poor relief could be much harsher. The able-bodied might be auctioned off as farm or other laborers in exchange for their keep. But even more significant for the future was the policy colonial towns adopted to differentiate among local and "strange" paupers, particularly after Britian started dumping "undesirables" on the colonies. Defining themselves as corporate entities with rights to decide whom they would welcome as permanent residents, colonial towns adopted a policy known as "warning out." While this policy permitted strangers to reside in the towns, it denied them poor relief. Such relief remained the responsibility of their home communities. But as war, industrialization, and other social and economic changes disrupted the normal small scale life of colonial towns and cities, poor relief also underwent changes.

Early adaptations to social change and to political disruption did not, in the beginning, fundamentally alter the traditional community response to the poor, the infirm, the insane, the old, and any other dependent person. Firmly embedded in communal and religious values buttressed by a shared pioneering experience, society remained in many ways deeply traditional. Old bonds of personal loyalties, born in the medieval past, persisted and fused the public and private. A shared religious framework for understanding and manipulating the world reinforced a society structured through webs of personal relationships (Wood, 1992). These religious and societal values not only sanctified hierarchy as innate but understood poverty and destitution as part of life's natural order (Rothman, 1971). Each person, however poor, counted for something in a great chain of existence. As long as communities could "warn out" strangers, their responsibility focused on their own. These features meant that relief policies could be integrated into the normal lives of individuals. The core moral values were, therefore, communal and reciprocal. Fostered by homogeneity and small, face-to-face communities, and, as yet untouched by urban individualism or industrialization, early American communities saw poverty and ill health as home-grown, familiar, and not morally blameworthy. Decision makers were local leaders; the poor had names and faces.

From Poor Relief to Almshouses: An Era of Optimism, 1820 to 1865

These values did not survive the rapid changes that overtook American society. Even in the mid-eighteenth century, a demographic explosion and economic changes unsettled old patterns and values. Commercial capitalism inserted the cash nexus into formerly hierarchically determined personal relationships (Wood, 1992). The revolution itself sharply—and, as it turned out, irrevocably—challenged every form of authority and superiority (Wood, 1992), including the religious. Change in almost every aspect of American life was endemic, rapid, and interactive as the nineteenth century dawned. Relief policies inevitably shifted.

The most visible result was a deepening preference for "indoor" rather than "outdoor" relief, a watershed in social welfare policy. Although larger cities had started housing vagrants and some older people in almshouses as early as the seventeenth century, by the eighteenth century that trend had deepened. Still a place of last resort, an occasionally necessary and nonstigmatizing substitute household, particularly for its older inmates, the almshouse was maintained by charitable contributions and neighborhood volunteers (Butners, 1980; Rothman, 1971) for those who could not be cared for in their own homes or in the homes of neighbors. From the 1820s forward, in contrast, almshouses became the preferred form of public support in most communities for all dependent populations, including the elderly; they joined other institutions—prisons, mental hospitals, and orphan asylums—as deliberate instruments of social policy.

Early nineteenth-century reformers, focusing almost single-mindedly on the individual, optimistically believed that they could cure all that ailed society. As the diversity of communities accelerated, however, they faced poor and infirm individuals who were not always friends, neighbors, relatives, or "worthy" English, especially widows, and as the need for labor gradually eroded the "warning out" policies, the *Gemeinschaft* character of small preindustrial communities yielded to ethnically and increasingly racially diverse towns and cities (Kutzik, 1979). These changes roused fears of disorder and ruptured the strong bonds that linked poor relief to religious, hierarchical, and communal values.

As early as 1817, attacks on "foreign paupers" deepened; by the 1820s and 1830s the language of poor relief became harsher and strident (Kutzik, 1979). Although some paupers were still deemed worthy, more and more were castigated as depraved and vicious (Rothman, 1971). Whatever other explanations seem salient, the surge in European immigration provoked a nativist response and significantly influenced the tilt toward institutional care (Quadagno, 1986).

When the young nation experienced its first depression from 1817 to 1821, an escalating poor tax, triggered by the sharp elevation in poverty, made poor relief the object of study. The institutional solution emerged as a clear favorite. In New York, the influential Yates Report, published in 1824, established the principles of "indoor" relief in New York State. The Yates Report led to the County Poorhouse Act of 1824, which made the county poorhouse the center of public relief (Butners, 1980). In Philadelphia, public "outdoor" relief ended in the 1830s to be replaced by almshouses (Kutzik, 1979). In the early decades of the nineteenth century, so many states passed legislation comparable to New York's that by 1857 the treatment of poverty had become synonymous with the almshouse (Rothman, 1971). First in the East and then in the Middle West and Far West, "indoor" relief replaced "outdoor" relief. By mid-century, most poor and infirm older people, who needed assistance beyond what family or neighbors could offer, had few choices but the almshouse.

Yet something other than convenience, cost-effectiveness, and even nativist sentiment predisposed the investigators to view the institutional solution so favorably. To optimistic Jacksonian Democrats of the 1820s, accepting poverty as part of life's natural order was unacceptable. Feeling compelled to explain rather than accept poverty, reformers frequently concluded that "economic failure was due to moral failure" (Rothman, 1971, p. 162). The Quincy Report, issued in Massachusetts in 1821, argued that "of all causes of pauperism, intemperance, in the use of spirituous liquors, is the most powerful and universal" (Rothman, 1971, p. 163). Evidence of indolence, intemperance, and other vices strengthened reformers' claim that the poor required moral elevation; in particular, they had to be saved from behaviors that caused socially corrosive pauperism. This reforming zealotry located the causes of poverty in the individual; the poor were to be saved from themselves.

Filled with a sense of moral urgency, middle-class, Protestant reformers labored to make "others" over in their own image. They commonly used morals testing to justify supervision of those they assisted and to divide the "worthy" from the "unworthy" poor (Gordon, 1991). Modern policies, for example, Medicare and Medicaid, bear the marks of this distinction. So do current debates about paternalism and attitudes toward reciprocity. As the newly consolidating professional classes, such as physicians and social workers, defined poverty in terms of moral laxity if not depravity, paternalistic interventions reigned unchecked. At the same time, the grounds for social reciprocity disappeared. If the poor were morally depraved, they had little to offer others. Instead they became moral children, expected not to choose but to obey. By midcentury, the reformers' zealousness for social improvement accelerated the growth of specialized institutions designed to reform, rehabilitate, and educate.

These attitudes, buttressed by the large numbers of urban and foreign-born poor, distorted the original communal goal of relief practices: to ease misery. Poor relief administrators had an additional task—to reconcile compassion with the need to "deter people from relying on public and private relief" (Katz, 1984, p. 115). Although many reformers thought of the almshouses optimistically, as a way "to help the genuinely needy from starving without breeding a class of paupers" (Katz, 1984, p. 114), one solution was to make relief so unpleasant that few would opt for it. Deliberately punitive, the poorhouse was meant to enforce discipline and motivate individuals to lead upstanding lives. Poorhouses were also intended to regulate labor markets by creating a forced choice between low wages and the poorhouse. Hence, the threat of the poorhouse served capital in a way that the more benign "outdoor" relief could not (Katz, 1984).

With the growth of urban and immigrant poverty and the new ideology of self-reliance, attitudes toward illness and dependency in old age began to shift. Until the middle third of the nineteenth century, many Americans still accepted sickness and dependency as inevitable dimensions of growing old. In contrast, Victorian moralists came to devalue those who experienced poverty, disease, and frailty in old age. Viewing these conditions as signs of personal moral failure, health reformers and ministers believed that aging well, like the rest of life, was within individual control (Cole, 1992). This belief was thus mapped onto older people; not unexpectedly, this dichotomy often translated directly into "worthy" native-born American women versus unworthy "others." Blinded to the social and economic causes of poverty and ill health, many reformers blamed poor men for profligacy and immigrants for slovenly work habits and other non-Protestant characteristics.

Shocked to discover the presence of white native-born, and therefore "worthy" women in the almshouses, poor by no fault of their own, white Protestant reformers developed private homes for the aged, for those of appropriate caste and nativity (Butners, 1980). As early as 1814, the Association for the Relief of Respectable Aged Indigent Females was founded in New York City. It erected its first "asylum" in 1838 (Cole, 1985). With comparable motives, in 1817 Philadelphians founded the Indigent Widows' and Single Women's Society, which denied admission to anyone born and raised in poverty. In that same city, but 50 years later, the Quakers and African-Americans opened the doors to a home for "worthy and exemplary colored people," in recognition that racism and not bad character had made them poor (Haber, 1983, pp. 101 and 102). Comparable homes were founded in many other cities to care for people who became poor not because of bad character but as the result of fickle fortune.

White Protestant reformers were not alone in their efforts to create alternatives to the almshouse. Under varied auspices, private efforts—modest by today's standards—supplemented public welfare. As the number of almshouses grew and charity became more punitive, ethnic and racial minorities began systematic efforts to assist their own (Kutzik, 1979). According to W.E.B. DuBois (1909), the establishment of old people's homes was the "most characteristic Negro charity" (p. 65) in the postbellum period. Homes for the aged, often sponsored by women's organizations, were soon founded in a number of cities. "Negroes," especially in the South, also sought to fill voids left by government neglect (Rabinowitz, 1974).

Although not new to the early nineteenth century, these mutual aid societies greatly expanded their memberships and the diversity of their sponsorship. Like colonial poor relief, by helping families through rough times, they also facilitated family support of older family members. Although immigrants from Scotland formed the first mutual aid societies, by the middle of the nineteenth century, Jewish and African-American organizations dominated the field. Among free African-Americans in Philadelphia, for example, deteriorating race relations, economic depression, and the resulting inaccessibility of white English public assistance and organized charity "strengthened already strong motivations for Blacks to care for themselves" (Kutzik, 1979, p. 41). In the South, a number of benevolent societies were founded. In Atlanta, one benevolent society's motto stated that "We assist the needy; we relieve our sick; we bury our dead" (Rabinowitz, 1974, p. 338). This pattern of mutual aid and reliance on the black community for providing and subsidizing social services survived vigorously until the ravages of the depression threatened their already fragile economic condition and diminished, without eliminating, their ability to assist families (McRoy, 1990).

The Decline of the Poorhouse and the Road to Social Security: 1865 to 1935

In an ironic twist, older people between 1865 and 1935 became the "natural" and principal inhabitants of the almshouse, created initially to save money, to reform the able-bodied poor, and to meet other less benign social goals. At first by chance, the result of policies designed for other population groups (see below), and later as a deliberate social goal, the almshouse became an old-age home.

From 1830 to 1850, people over 50 constituted 18 percent of the population in northeastern almshouses. From 1880 to 1920, the national proportion of almshouse residents who were old rose from 33 percent to 66 percent, most of them foreign-born (Haber and Gratton, 1993; Cole, 1992). Not surprisingly, after midcentury, the ties between a dependent older population and the almshouse became ingrained in the American mind. Older people were also the dominant recipients of "outdoor" relief. In 1826, 61 percent of those on outdoor relief in Philadelphia were over 50; by 1929 that figure had risen to 80 percent (Quadagno, 1986).

The graying of the almshouse population in the second half of the nineteenth century occurred by default, not because so many more older individuals became disabled or poor. "Outdoor" relief, deemed too expensive, became less available. More systematically than earlier in the century, reformers moved specific groups into separate institutions (Katz, 1986). The young went to orphanages, the insane to mental institutions, the physically handicapped to special schools, and the able-bodied to workhouses (Haber, 1983). Imbued with the Progressive ideology of social reform, reformers focused on classification and reform—but not for old people. Because physicians held little hope for ameliorating the pathological conditions of old age, old people were rarely transferred to other institutions (Haber and Gratton, 1994).

By stripping away one group after another, these reformers unintentionally, but nonetheless effectively, transformed the almshouse into a residence for older, poor people (Katz, 1984). External forces also drove more and more older people into almshouses. Many private charities, for example, declined to assist the old whom they considered "nonredeemable" and therefore permanently dependent (Haber and Gratton, 1994; Quadagno, 1986). As medical science became more curative, hospitals became less willing to serve as custodial institutions, and hospital administrators wanted the old who consumed beds and resources that could be put to "better" use removed from their facilities (Haber, 1983; Rosenberg, 1987).

By the late nineteenth century, hospitals increasingly resisted admitting the old and the chronically impaired, arguing that the old should receive medical care but preferably not in private medical facilities or even state mental institutions because they could no longer benefit from real assistance (Haber and Gratton, 1994; Haber, 1983). Thus, the physically and mentally infirm were moved to almshouses or to municipal hospitals. By these varied routes, the almshouse, not initially designed to house older people as the primary residents, became their "home," a home that was also increasingly custodial and soon also medicalized. The almshouses became the rough equivalents of modern public nursing homes and chronic care facilities.

As the above suggests, the institutional solution to problems of dependence did not arise from the decline of family support. Close and instrumental kinship relationships persisted through most of this history. Contrary to earlier assumptions, industrialization did not represent a sharp disruption in family ties. Instead, families seem to have maintained a high degree of structural integrity (Seward, 1978), honoring two cultural norms: family responsibility and autonomous living (Haber and Gratton, 1994). Thus, although the percentages and absolute numbers of older people in almshouses climbed, the decline of family support was not one of the reasons for the rise.

In the last decades of the nineteenth century, conditions in the almshouses generally worsened. Financial problems were only one source of the difficulties. Again the conflict between compassion and deterrence played an important role. Some reformers, such as members of the State Charities Aid Association founded in 1872 and the Charity Organization Society founded in 1881, began to rethink almshouse policies especially for the "worthy" aged. But they were never able to reconcile the conflicting purposes of the almshouses. Still focused on the individual, the charity reformers expressed concern about the "respectable" old woman whose sensitivity to how she differed from her fellow inmates earned her the right to otherwise unheard-of privacy (Clark, 1900). The reformers' concerns rarely resulted in significant change; perhaps they added a library or held religious services for those in the "terminal condition" of old age. The reformers expected all who could to work: to sew a rag rug, to wash the dishes, even if it had to be done sitting down

(Butners, 1980). Ironically, as nursing homes became more modern (and more medicalized), they also abandoned this earlier policy of responsibility and rough reciprocity.

Some late nineteenth century "scientific" reformers went further. They often used their power to campaign against all public welfare as the promoter of pauperism unless it had the singular aim of "curing" the individual (Butners, 1980). Even for the aged, they argued that better treatment would undermine filial responsibility; public welfare would weaken the social bonds necessary for a stable and orderly society. Although the aged did not wholly relinquish their "worthy" status to this group of reformers, old age dependency seemed closely tied to profligacy in youth. If not intemperate, the poor elderly were foolish and imprudent, not having saved for the proverbial rainy day (Rothman, 1971).

Nor were the aged free from nativist and paternalistic sentiment. In 1895, Mary Roberts Smith interviewed 228 women living in San Francisco's almshouse. She deemed nine worthy; all but one were native-born Americans. "The clearly honest, deserving, and unfortunate, because they are so few, stand out in sharp distinction to the mass of the degenerate and unworthy" (Smith, 1958, p. 258). The others—mostly foreign-born —deserved, in Smith's opinion, only minimal custodial care as penance for their earlier intemperate, immoral, and shiftless lives. Several years later, Smith recommended classifying inmates on the basis of their "habits, character, and degree of refinement" (Warner, 1908).

The late nineteenth century, then, was a period of serious deterioration in almshouses: minimal physical care, no recreation, no attention to emotional needs, and the separation of husbands and wives (Kutzik, 1979). Illness and insanity went untreated; filth and dilapidated conditions prevailed (Rothman, 1980). The early goals of the almshouse evaporated; custody replaced reform as the mainstay of institutional life. The poorhouse became a symbol of brutality and corruption (Cole, 1992). As the public grew more indifferent to the plight of the poor, withdrawing from an oversight role (Katz, 1984), the almshouses and their inhabitants were, in essence, abandoned.

The bad conditions in the almshouses and the increasing presence of older residents did not escape notice. In 1903, reformers like Homer Folks, New York's Commissioner of Charities, recommended, in an effort to lend dignity to older almshouse residents, that New York City's almshouse be renamed the Home for the Aged and Infirm. This name change did not radically alter care. Instead, it signified a changing perception of poverty and ill health in old age. Folks argued that it was time to recognize that the "inmates of almshouses were more nearly related to hospital patients than paupers" (Haber and Gratton, 1994, p. 127). Backed by studies such as Mabel Louise Nassau's 1913 study of almshouses, public welfare reformers sought to remove the stigma of old-age poverty, blaming age itself as the source of problems. Though not returning full circle to the earlier Calvinist beliefs that dependence in old age is part of the human condition, these studies concluded that poverty often befell older men and women even when they had lived virtuously and worked hard all their lives (Cole, 1987). Supported by late nineteenth century medical investigations that combined pathology and old age, greater tolerance, if not respect, for old age poverty and ill health emerged. Aging itself became a disease, senility inevitable. Gone was the Victorian concept of self-willed health and independence. The new myth of old age, conforming to the late nineteenth century medical model of senescence, suggested that no matter how they lived, all old people would eventually become patients (Haber, 1983).

What once appeared a chance occurrence, the burgeoning population of elder almshouse residents, was now touted as the best setting to care for the impoverished and incapacitated elderly (Haber, 1983). Using a model of old-age dependency, scientific charity reformers vigorously advocated for the institution as the appropriate place to care for the sick elderly; the almshouse gained a new status in the annals of scientific charity. In the eyes of the reformers, it became the location of choice for the severely incapacitated aged of limited means or even competent but poor elders (Haber, 1983; Kutzik, 1979).

This attitude also encouraged the continued establishment of private old-age homes. According to many professionals, the institution was the residence of choice to meet an older person's inevitable medical needs. As needs for medical care grew, institutional facilities added nursing staff and evolved into the now familiar nursing home or personal care homes with infirmaries (Dunlop, 1979). By the early twentieth century, more than 1000 private homes for the aged were in the United States (Pegels, 1988).

Even the almshouse became more hospital-like. For most needy older people, the almshouse, the linchpin of the public welfare system into the twentieth century, was their source of care. Care of the indigent elderly had become the basic function of the nation's poorhouses. Long-term care for the aged poor, regardless of their mental condition, meant almshouse residency (Haber and Gratton, 1994).

Nineteenth-century social welfare policies, rendered visible in alms-houses, and to a lesser extent in private homes for the aged, reveal the links between ideology and behavior. The consequences for older people and their families were enormous. Because they were never the singular residents of almshouses, their fortunes inevitably varied with the more generalized social response to destitution, to America's "war on the able-bodied" poor (Katz, 1984, p. 115). They became victims of the authorities' antagonism to the idle, the intemperate, the poor, and the vicious, sharing living accommodations with society's most despised outcasts. They also fell victim to shifting definitions of their health, abilities, and prognosis, and to the vigorous efforts of groups to take care of their own (Haber and Gratton, 1994, pp. 122–139).

At the same time the almshouses also displayed the patterns of racial segregation that still persist in America's nursing homes. Needy African-Americans were either excluded from the almshouses or moved into the older facilities. In 1866, the first Negroes entered the old Nashville poor-house after extended negotiations between the municipality and the Freedman's Bureaus. As they arrived, white paupers relocated to new quarters (*Nashville Daily Press and Times,* April 13, 1867, cited in Rabi-nowitz, 1974).

These developments help us to understand contemporary ethical concerns for autonomy and decision making. Nowhere in the medical care system was there anything approximating the contemporary stress on patient autonomy, and for older patients, doubly harmed by poverty and ill health, decisional incapacity was often assumed. The residue of such cultural stereotypes is still visible in contemporary practice. Physicians often talk past the elder patient and address a family member; goals for the disabled elderly are ratcheted downward to focus on staying out of an institution (Cohen, 1988; Minkler, 1990), while autonomy is narrowly limited to what George Agich in Chapter 6 calls nodal decisions, and day-to-day autonomy is restricted by the demands of the institution.

From Social Security to the Present

Passage of the Social Security Act in 1935, although it directly addressed only the income side of the almshouses' dual function, nonetheless had a significant impact on the growth of institutional care. The added income from Social Security reduced the demand for custodial care as a result of pauperism. Instead older people did not enter a facility until their health deteriorated or family assistance was no longer available.

The result was a gradual transition to the private modern nursing home or personal care home. The Social Security Act severed the direct tie between poor relief and infirmity; it did not abolish the connection between class, race, ethnicity, and the kind of care an older person might obtain.

Although reformers such as New York's Homer Folks had argued for public, institutional provisions, the dismal record of and the social stigma associated with the almshouses steered the federal government in other directions. Its tool was the payment mechanism. The Social Security Act prohibited payments to residents of public homes, such as almshouses. The result was a substantial diminution in the use of public facilities until the 1950 Amendments to the Social Security Act changed this funding strategy. In the meanwhile, the number of private homes grew rapidly (Haber and Gratton, 1994) while public facilities remained, as they have to this day, the "care setting of last resort for the down-and-outer types . . . . [serving] the poorest but also some of the sickest nursing home patients" (Dunlop, 1977, p. 100).

From the 1930s to the 1960s, the modern nursing home, supported by federal legislation, took clearer shape as the singularly most important source of institutional care for America's elders. In 1940, 41 percent of institutionalized elders resided in a variety of group quarters—boarding homes and board and care facilities, for example; in 1970 the percentage had declined to 12 percent. In contrast, nursing home occupancy increased from 34 to 72 percent of all institutionalized persons in that same period. Services, however, remained meager. Thus, many chronically ill older persons continued to occupy beds in general hospitals. To free those beds for the more acutely ill, during the 1950s several federal programs encouraged the expansion of nursing homes.

This bias toward private, for-profit facilities encouraged by federal law had particularly important repercussions for African-Americans. Patterns of segregation led blacks to overcrowded county facilities, state-run mental hospitals, and unregulated personal care homes. The new nursing homes, like the older almshouses, were segregated. The passage, in 1965, of the Civil Rights Act and Title XVIII (Medicare) and Title XIX (Medicaid) of the Social Security Act did not substantially alter the historical pattern of segregation. Neither pressure from the Johnson administration nor the actions of regulators pushed nursing homes to integrate (Smith, 1979). In a much-quoted study, published in 1981, the Institute of Medicine (IOM) reported that ethnic/racial factors continued to influence the pattern of health care "in ways that are not in the interests of the groups affected . . . . a pattern of discrimination *seems* to be the cause" (p. 28). Although admitting that the evidence is scanty, the IOM concluded that "differences in access rather than ethnic social preferences account for most of the variation in user rates" (p. 87). Recent scholarship (Headen, 1992; Taylor, 1988) alerts us to avoid the easy assumption that African-American families do not use institutions *solely* because family support norms are so powerful. As Jacqueline Jones (1985) reminds us, in another context, "It is a cruel historical irony that scholars and policymakers alike have taken the manifestations of black women's oppression and twisted them into the argument that a powerful black matriarchy exists" (p. 7).

Conclusion

This dominant story, focused on the institutional components of long-term care, has had consequences far beyond the number of people it actually affected. For a generation old enough to remember, the almshouses represent the terrible stigma of public welfare. That stigma, rightly or wrongly, has been transferred to nursing homes.

By giving birth, albeit indirectly, to the private nursing home industry, the almshouse established the conditions that still separate low income elders from others. Reinforcing the invidious distinctions between the worthy and the unworthy poor, Medicaid reimbursement levels, combined with the commodification of care, contributed to dismal conditions that have made nursing homes among the most highly regulated institutions in modern society. These developments, in turn, have led to many structural constraints that impede the ethically sound decision making for which Agich (Chap. 6) and Bart Collopy (Chap. 7) argue. Yet, until recently ethicists have paid little attention to the structural constraints that impede actual autonomy and growth at the end of life.

Although it is a truism that each person experiences disability, illness, or poverty uniquely, public and social policy—directly and indirectly, by commission or omission—treats individuals according to their status in a broader social group. For most of their history, the old belonged to the group known as the poor. In the last decades of the nineteenth century, when social reformers identified the elderly as a group requiring specialized attention, they understood old age in negative terms. Today, that context is shifting; older people and their advocates are emphasizing the positive aspects of old age. Future historians will reflect how this new image, when combined with fiscal austerity and "granny bashing," manifests more general social patterns.

In closing, it is important to reaffirm that the centrality of institutions in the story of long-term care obscures important factors. Most older people continue to live independently, requiring little help apart from occasional services that families normally exchange on a daily basis and in times of emergency (Brody and Brody, 1989). When help is needed, the family is still the first line of defense. Though a detailed account is beyond the scope of this essay, it must still be noted that the pattern and burden of family caregiving are neither uniform nor divorced from external realities. In particular, patterns of discrimination and socioeconomic status have severely constrained the choices available to African-American families. Oppression, institutional racism, and economic deprivation forced black families to adapt with great creativity. Thus, black elders can substitute one type of informal helper for another if a spouse or a child is no longer available (Gibson and Jackson, 1987).

These often hidden, often courageous parallel stories, the ones that took place in families and neighborhoods, have had little influence, until recently, on public policy or on the way American society constructed its image of old-age dependency. Although contemporary gerontology is finely attuned to the family's role as the primary source of long-term care, mainstream bioethics has tended to overlook that interdependency and its ethical implications. John Arras discusses these implications in Chapter 10. The locus of interest has been the individual. In what may be another watershed, the growing expectation by nursing homes that older people will have executed advance directives may, once again, limit choices. In part an appropriate reaction to the history just described, this approach arguably ignores the central fact in the lives of many elders—that they are part of families. The risk is that, once again, families will be given less than their due. For this reason, considerations such as those developed by Nancy Jecker (Chap. 8), Sarah Brakman (Chap. 9), and John Arras (Chap. 10) compel attention. In addition, taking the family seriously also suggests that forms of decision making not requiring advance directives remain available.

Ideologies, whether religious, scientific, or medical, along with race, ethnicity, class, and gender, dramatically shaped—and still shape—long-term care for the aged. Any society or culture constructs old age and aging through a web of institutional structures and cultural meanings.

Throughout its history long-term care mediated many intersections among individuals, families, and society. Similarly, study of the microworld of the institution reveals the larger institutional and social forces that structure the experience of old age. Our account reflects the shifting historiography of both old age and the family and illuminates the relationships among older people, social and economic organization, and ideology.

NOTES

1. We use the term ideology in a sense common among historians: as a set of beliefs (not necessarily true or false) that represent the world view or self-interest of a certain group of people.

2. Like the English poor law system from which it derived, early American poor relief had no separate institutional structure. It was, therefore, known as outdoor relief. The first separate institutional provisions for poor relief, known as the almshouse or the poorhouse, came to be known as indoor relief (see Quadagno, 1988).

REFERENCES

Benjamin, A.E. (1993). An historical perspective on home care policy. *Milbank Quarterly, 71*: 129–166.

Berkhofer, R. (1989). The challenge of poetics to (normal) historical practice. In P. Hernadi (ed.), *The Rhetoric of Interpretation and the Interpretation of Rhetoric*, pp. 183–200. Durham, N.C.: Duke University Press.

Brody, E.M., and Brody, S.J. (1989). The informal system of health care. In C. Eisdorfer, P.A. Kessler, and A.N. Spector (eds.), *Caring for the Elderly: Reshaping Health Care Policy*, pp. 259–277. Baltimore: Johns Hopkins University Press.

Butners, A. (1980). *Institutionalized Altruism and the Aged: Charitable Provision for the Aged in New York City, 1865–1930*. Ph.D. diss., Columbia University, New York.

Clark, M.V. (1900). The almshouse. In *Proceedings of the National Conference of Charities and Corrections.*

Cohen, E. (1988). The elderly mystique: Constraints on the autonomy of the elderly with disabilities. *Gerontologist, 28*(Supplement): 24–31.

Cole, T. (1985). Aging and meaning: Our society provides no compelling answers. *Generations, 10*: 49–52.

Cole, T. (1987). Class, culture, and coercion: A historical perspective on longterm care. *Generations, 11*: 9–15.

Cole, T. (1992). *Journey of Life*. New York: Cambridge University Press.

Dowling, H. (1982). *The City Hospitals: The Undercare of the Underprivileged*. Cambridge: Harvard University Press.

DuBois, W.E.B. (1909). *The Social Betterment among Negro Americans*. Atlanta: Atlanta University Press.

Dunlop. B.D. (1979). *The Growth of Nursing Home Care*. Lexington, Mass.: Lexington Books.

Gibson, R., and Jackson, J. (1987). The health, physical functioning, and informal supports of the black elderly. *Milbank Quarterly, 65*(Supplement 2): 421–454.

Gordon, L. (1991). Black and white visions of welfare: Women's welfare activism, 1890–1945. *Journal of American History, 78*: 559–590.

Haber, C. (1983). *Beyond Sixty-five*. New York: Cambridge University Press.

Haber, C., and Gratton, B. (1994). *Old Age and the Search for Security: An American Social History*. Bloomington, Ind.: Indiana University Press.

Headen, A.E. (1992). Time costs and informal social supports as determinants of differences between black and white families in the provision of long-term care. *Inquiry, 29*: 440–450.

Institute of Medicine. (1981). *Health Care in the Context of Civil Rights*. Washington, D.C.: National Academy Press.

Jones, J. (1985). *Labor of Love, Labor of Sorrow*. New York: Basic Books.

Katz, M. (1984). Poorhouses and the origins of public old age homes. *Milbank Memorial Quarterly/Health and Society, 62*: 110–140.

Katz, M. (1986). *In the Shadow of the Poorhouse*. New York: Basic Books.

Kutzik, A. (1979). American social provision for the aged: An historical perspective. In D. Gelfand and A. Kutzik (eds.), *Ethnicity and Aging: Theory, Research, and Policy*, pp. 32–65. New York: Springer Publishing Co.

McClure, E. (1968). *More Than a Roof: The Development of Minnesota Poor Farms and Homes for the Aged*. St. Paul, Minn.: Minnesota Historical Society.

McRoy, R.G. (1990). A historical overview of black families. In S. Logan, E. Freeman, and R. McRoy (eds.), *Social Work Practice with Black Families*, pp. 3–17. White Plains, N.Y.: Longman.

Minkler, M. (1990). Aging and disability: Behind and beyond the stereotypes. *Journal of Aging Studies, 4*: 245–260.

Nashville Daily Press and Times (April 13, 1867), quoted in Rabinowitz, H.N. (1974). From exclusion to segregation: Health and welfare services for southern blacks. *Social Services Review, 48*: 327–354.

Okin, S.M. (1989). *Justice, Gender, and the Family*. New York: Basic Books.

Pegels, C. (1988). *Health Care and the Older Citizen: Economic, Demographic, and Financial Aspects.* Rockville, Md.: Aspen Systems.

Quadagno, J. (1986). The transformation of old age security. In D. Van Tassel and P. Stearns (eds.), *Old Age in a Bureaucratic Society,* pp. 129–155. New York: Greenwood Press.

Quadagno, J. (1988). *The Transformation of Old Age Security.* Chicago: University of Chicago Press.

Rabinowitz, H.N. (1974). From exclusion to segregation: Health and welfare services for southern blacks. *Social Services Review, 48:* 327–354.

Rosenberg, C. (1987). *The Care of Strangers: The Rise of America's Hospital System.* New York: Basic Books.

Rothman, D. (1971). *The Discovery of the Asylum.* Boston: Little, Brown and Co.

Rothman, D. (1980). *Conscience and Convenience: The Asylum and Its Alternative in Progressive America.* Boston: Little, Brown and Co.

Seward, R. (1978). *The American Family: A Demographic History.* Beverly Hills, Calif.: Sage Publications.

Smith, D.S. (1979). Life course, norms, and the family system of older Americans in 1900. *Journal of Family History, 4:* 285–298.

Smith, M.R. (1895). Almshouse women: A study of two hundred and twenty-eight women in the city and county almshouse of San Francisco. *American Statistical Association, 8:* 258.

Taylor, R.J. (1988). Aging and supportive relationships among black Americans. In J. Jackson (ed.), *The Black American Elderly: Research on Physical and Psychosocial Health,* pp. 259–281. New York: Springer Publishing Co.

Warner, A. (1908). *American Charities.* New York: Thomas Crowell Co.

Wood, G. (1992). *The Radicalism of the American Revolution.* New York: Alfred A. Knopf.

CHAPTER THREE

Long-Term Care in the United States: An Overview of the Current System

Nancy L. Wilson

The professional literature, public media, and public policy discussions are giving increased attention to long-term care. For several reasons American society now recognizes a new situation: the survival of large numbers of severely disabled persons at a time when most adults, including women, the traditional caregivers in the United States, are employed. Demographic trends, with which most of us are familiar, show significant growth in the old-old population (persons older than 75), who have a high prevalence of functional impairment and chronic disease. The increased pressure on public expenditures for nursing home care and other long-term care services concerns the makers of public policy. Disabled individuals and their family members face daily worries about coping with disability, maintaining self-identity and family identity, and adjusting financial and time budgets to the burdens of chronic disease that may last indefinitely. The dialogue on long-term care is also fueled by the fact that "in an era of overall health care reform, indeed, no other part of the health care system generates as much passionate dissatisfaction as long-term care" (Wiener and Hixon Illston, 1994).

Over the past decade, the authors of many important books and articles on long-term care (among them Ory and Duncker, 1992; Kane and Kane, 1987; Kemper, Applebaum, and Harrigan, 1987; Brody and Magel, 1989; Harrington, Newcomer, and Estes, 1985; Leutz et al., 1992; Rivlin and Wiener, 1988; Estes, Swan, and Associates, 1993) have addressed policy options and advanced recommendations for improving the organization, delivery, and financing of long-term care. This chapter is intended to provide some basic understanding of the current status of long-term care in the United States. This includes current definitions of long-term care, the older client population needing long-term care services, and approaches to the financing, organization, and delivery of services.

Although it is the elderly, especially the very old, who typically need long-term care, people of any age might experience physical or mental limitations that require them to have long-term care. Individuals with developmental disabilities, for example, or those with chronic mental illness and other chronic disease may need such care. The discussions in this volume are limited, however, to the long-term care needs of older people, who, as they age, are particularly susceptible to chronic conditions that lead to permanent functional disability and, as Terrie Wetle discusses in Chapter 4, are often at particular ethical risk in social policy decisions.

Defining Long-Term Care

Long-term care is defined in many different ways. A comprehensive definition is provided by Rosalie and Robert Kane (Kane and Kane, 1987): "Long-term care is a set of health, personal care, and social services delivered over a sustained period of time to persons who have lost or never acquired some degree of functional capacity" (p. 4). For many people long-term care is often equated with the settings in which it is given or with the programs that provide a specific service. To many people, long-term care means nursing homes because this is where most long-term care public dollars are spent. The conceptual definition of long-term care focuses not, however, on the place where services are offered, but on the help that compensates for functional problems. As Kane and Kane (1987) noted, long-term care sits uncomfortably on the boundary between health and social services and includes elements of both. Furthermore, because of health conditions that may produce or complicate a person's functional disability, a person receiving long-term care must also rely on acute-care services. As many scholars have noted, there must be careful "orchestration" between acute- and long-term care programs, and often the lines between the two are drawn by the financing system and not by the needs of the population concerned (Kane and Kane, 1987, 1989; Leutz et al., 1992).

The close link between medical conditions that produce disability and the continuing need for care has contributed a further distinction in the definition of long-term care. The services intended to address the needs of the temporarily needy (i.e., care needed less than ninety days) frail elderly were characterized as "short-term long-term care" by Stanley Brody and Judith Magel (1984) and as postacute care by Kane and Kane (1990). Under this distinction, "long-term long-term care" (Brody and Magel, 1984) refers to services required over an indefinite if not continuous period by individuals who have permanent functional limitations. Another important distinction in understanding long-term care concerns service setting. Long-term care services to persons with functional limitations can be delivered in an institution, in a home or residence, or in what is referred to as a community setting.

The Population Needing Long-Term Care

Activities of daily living are being commonly used as a broad measure of long-term care needs in research, policy making, and practice (Stone and Murtaugh, 1990). The term *activities of daily living* (ADL) refers to an individual's ability to accomplish such personal care tasks as toileting, bathing, and dressing. Another common measure concerns a person's ability to perform such instrumental activities of daily living (IADL) as meal preparation, shopping, and money management.

Because long-term care is increasingly defined on the basis of the population served, it is important to understand the diverse older client population in need of long-term care. The following three portraits of real situations (with names changed) and other cases discussed in this book (see Collopy, Chap. 7; Jecker, Chap. 8; and Arras, Chap. 10) illustrate some of the diverse needs and disparate resources of the long-term care population.

CASE I

Joseph Weinbrach is a 90-year-old married man who has multiple functional deficits caused by dementia, Parkinson's disease, and previous cerebrovascular accidents. He lives at home with his 81-year-old wife of fifty-nine years who is obese, hypertensive, and has severe osteoarthritis of the knees, hips, and spine. Because of her health problems, Janet Weinbrach has difficulty walking, and she has never driven a car. She has been her husband's full-time caregiver for the past nine years, and she also cared for their 51-year-old daughter before the daughter's death from emphysema. The family's income is less than $1200 a month with their other assets quite limited, which is why Mrs. Weinbrach receives thirty hours a week of publicly financed help with household tasks and her husband's personal care. Their two remaining children live out-of-state, but they do as much as they can to ease their parents' financial needs, including money management and buying prescription drugs. Mrs. Weinbrach still treasures her husband's company and despite her circumstances wishes to continue to be his primary provider. Mr. Weinbrach's brief stay in a nursing facility following one of his hospital stays left his wife very dissatisfied with the option of institutional care.

CASE 2

Louise James is a 77-year-old widow whose medical problems include congestive heart failure, arthritis, and right-leg amputation below the knee made necessary by complications from slow-healing leg ulcers. Following a short rehabilitation stay in a skilled nursing facility after her amputation, Mrs. James again lives alone in a rented house, relying for financial support on Social Security and a small pension from her previous employment with the school district. Her confinement to a wheelchair and other health problems make it necessary for her to have help with bathing and many home maintenance tasks. Her home has several architectural barriers that limit her mobility, but her neighborhood includes many longstanding friends. Despite her disability, she wants to continue living alone and is currently receiving some services through her Medicare home health benefits. Her only daughter is employed and provides regular assistance to her mother, including meal preparation and all of her mother's shopping and errands that require transportation. Neighbors and friends also help as much as they can.

CASE 3

Mrs. West is a 91-year-old widowed woman who has had a stroke that left her paralyzed on the left side and unable to transfer herself from bed to chair independently. She cannot do most ADLs without assistance. Her twenty-four-hour need for help has caused her to leave her neighborhood and move in with her 70-year-old divorced daughter. She attends privately financed adult day care so that her daughter can continue to work for their joint household and contribute to the costs of her mother's care.

How common are these needs and care arrangements, and how do these brief descriptions typify some of the client subgroups who need long-term care? Although surviving to old age does not guarantee that one will require long-term care, recent research has increased our understanding of long-term care as a "normal risk of growing old" (Wiener, 1990, p. 5) As Martha Holstein and Thomas Cole note in this volume (Chap. 2), the overwhelming majority of older people do not face signif-

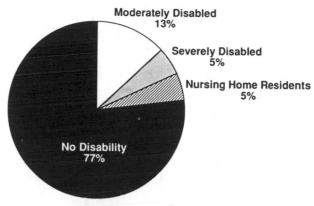

Figure 1. Distribution of the population aged 65 and older by extent of disability, 1989. *Source:* Modified from Rowland and Lyons (1991).

icant disability on any given day. Increased longevity, however, raises the likelihood of functional disability. Figure 1 shows the distribution of the population aged 65 and older by the extent of disability, based on data analyzed from the 1982 National Long-Term Care Survey (Rowland and Lyons, 1991, p. 4).

As the data in Figure 1 show, physical or cognitive disability affects one in four of older Americans sixty-five and older, including persons requiring nursing home care. The category of moderate disability shown in the chart includes individuals with one ADL limitation who need direct human assistance or require special equipment and those who need, on a standby basis, another person to help them perform one or more activities they cannot do themselves. This information illustrates the commonly cited fact that for every functionally disabled individual in a nursing home, two to three individuals with limitations are residing in the community.

As Peter Kemper and Christopher Murtaugh wrote in 1991, of those turning 65 in 1990, about 43 percent would enter a nursing home at some time before they died. Of those entering nursing homes, 55 percent would spend at least one year and 21 percent at least five years or more in the nursing home. Gender and ethnic status, however, affect nursing home use significantly (Kemper and Murtaugh, 1991). Projections for persons reaching age 65 in 1990 indicated that one in three women would spend at least one year in a nursing home, whereas only one in seven men would do so. Adjusting for differences in longevity and gen-

Table 1. Functionally Dependent Persons 65 Years Old and Older

	Type of Long-Term Care				Living Arrangements				
Dependency Level	All Types of Long-Term Care	Nursing Home Care	Formal Home Care	Informal Home Care	Total	Alone	Living with Spouse	Living with Others	Living Nursing Home
	Percentage Distribution					Percentage Distribution			
Totally dependent in ADL or IADL	79.0	16.4	20.6	42.0	100.0	28.7	35.7	19.2	16.4
5–7 ADL dependencies	100.0	59.1	16.4	24.5	100.0	4.7	18.7	17.4	59.1
3–4 ADL dependencies	100.0	25.9	22.8	51.3	100.0	11.8	33.5	28.9	25.9
1–2 ADL dependencies	62.4	6.0	15.8	40.6	100.0	34.6	41.2	18.2	6.0
Dependent in IADL only	90.0	4.0	32.5	53.5	100.0	39.8	37.3	18.9	4.0

Source: Modified from Hing (1990). Data from the 1984 National Health Interview Survey.

der between whites and African-Americans, a much higher percentage of whites than African-Americans use nursing homes. Likewise, elders of all four nonwhite categories—Asian-Pacific islanders, African-Americans, Hispanics, and Native Americans—are significantly underrepresented in the U.S. nursing home population despite evidence of greater disability in most of these populations (Yeo, 1993).

The information in Table 1 further defines the circumstances of the elderly long-term care population by showing individuals according to subgroups formed according to level of dependence in IADL or ADL (Hing, 1990, pp. 8 and 12). *Types* of long-term care refer to help the person is receiving from a family member or friend (informal home care), one or more paid providers (formal home care), or in an institution (nursing home care).

A key dimension of long-term care service delivery is the living arrangement of the person requiring assistance. Kovar (1988) identified a progression of dependence, as a result of increasing disability in the living arrangements of the elderly, beginning with living alone, then with other people (if possible), to living in a nursing home. The particularly significant role of spousal caregivers is highlighted in the living arrangements of persons who, having five to seven ADL disabilities, are almost totally dependent. The importance of examining the meaning of marriage in old age, as Nancy Jecker does in this volume (Chap. 8), is underscored by the fact that living with a spouse is currently the most common arrangement among elderly with IADL or ADL dependence. Joseph and Janet Weinbrach are typical of many people in long-term care situations in which community living remains possible because of a spousal caregiver whose own health may be affected by caregiving duties. Like Mr. Weinbrach, Louise James has more than one medical problem that contributes to her need for help. Their health is so unstable that either one may periodically require medical treatment at home or in a hospital. Overall use of health care services is greater among the functionally dependent population (Hing, 1990). Mrs. James, widowed like most women over 75 and living alone with multiple ADL disabilities, is at particular risk of having to enter a nursing home, as is reflected in the small percentage of persons living alone with three or more ADL dependencies. Mrs. James and Mrs. West depend heavily on their adult children, in both cases daughters who are employed outside the home but who provide essential assistance to enable their mothers to remain at home. Mrs. West and her 70-year-old daughter represent the growing number of families with more than one generation older than 65.

In terms of functional needs and health status as well as personal, social, and economic resources, the long-term care population is highly diverse. Some high-risk groups can be identified, however, according to sociodemographic factors. Compared with the total population 65 and older, the disabled elderly are disproportionately more likely to be women, aged 85 and older, and poor. Persons who are severely disabled (by two or more ADL limitations) are also more likely to belong to a minority race. Because of the important role of family members in maintaining disabled adults in the community, individuals without close family members are statistically overrepresented in the nursing home population. Specifically, widows, widowers, and those who have never married or are divorced or separated are most likely to be residents of nursing homes. Because of their longer life expectancy and tendency to outlive their spouses, older women are most likely to be represented in the nursing home population.

The size of the long-term care population in the United States varies, depending on the definition of functional impairment used (i.e., the number of ADLs or IADLs included), the methods of measurement, as well as such other factors as age and income that may be applied to define the population (Rowland et al., 1988). Many states use measures of ADL only to establish service eligibility; in current proposals before Congress, including the Clinton Health Security Act, ADLs are used as eligibility criteria for long-term care. According to the Clinton Health Security Act, the population eligible for services would include persons who (a) need help in the performance of three or more activities of daily living, (b) have severe cognitive or mental impairment or mental retardation, and (c) are children under the age of six who otherwise would be institutionalized. This definition of eligibility would make an estimated 3.1 million persons eligible for long-term care, and of that group 71 percent would be older persons (Oriol, 1993).

Apart from the obvious fiscal implications of targeting services to a narrowly or broadly defined impaired population, other issues arise, including how the provision of publicly supported services would affect the continued involvement of family caregivers.

The Role of Family in Long-Term Care

Consensus may be lacking on the best operational definition of the long-term care population, but the fact that the primary providers of long-term care are family members is undisputed. Most disabled older people live with one or more family members (Table 1). Holstein and Cole (Chap. 2) and Elaine and Steve Brody chronicle the situation: "The family invented long-term care of the elderly well before that phrase was articulated. . . . The family has always been and continues to be the main provider of long-term health and social support to the aged" (Brody and Brody, 1989, p. 259). Research done over several years indicates that not only do families provide most long-term care, today they provide more care and more difficult care to larger numbers of old people over longer time periods than ever before (Brody and Brody, 1989, p. 271). Liu and colleagues (1985) reported that almost three-quarters of disabled old people living outside institutions rely solely on unpaid help from family members and, to a lesser extent, friends and neighbors. Furthermore, as illustrated by the three cases discussed earlier, the overwhelming majority of persons receiving formal care are also helped informally by others. Comparable national information for the nursing home population is not available, but the indications are that many older nursing home residents continue to receive care from family members (George and Maddox, 1989). Moreover, the level of informal care the disabled elderly person receives increases with his or her disability at a much higher rate than does formal care under the same circumstances (Kemper, 1992).

A national profile of family members who provide long-term care reveals that adult children are most frequently the primary caregivers, followed by spouses, siblings, and other relatives. Irrespective of relationship to the care receiver, most of these caregivers are women who have been providing assistance for one to four years, almost 20 percent having provided care for five years or more (Stone, Cafferata, and Sangl, 1987). Like Mrs. Weinbrach, many of the caregivers are themselves old (35 percent over age 65), and like Mrs. West's daughter, about one third are working outside the home (Stone, Cafferata, and Sangl, 1987).

In recent years the costs of caregiving have been examined extensively. One obvious inequity is that women bear the disproportionate share of the uncompensated cost of providing informal care. Although a husband may be involved in the care of an older spouse, older women are more likely to assume this role because women are more likely to outlive their husbands. Like Mrs. Weinbrach, many spousal caregivers may suffer some of the consequences documented in studies of caregiving, including isolation, economic hardship, physical health problems, and low morale (Horowitz, 1985). The principal caregivers to dependent parents and parents-in-law are daughters and to some extent daughters-in-law. Elaine Brody, a pioneer in studies of family care, has noted that parent care is now a normative experience for individuals in families despite the increasing demands of responsibility for their own children and the growing participation of women in the work force (Brody, 1985). Although the majority of caregiving women are between the ages of 40 and 60, a significant number of those under 40 and over 60 face unique challenges because of their own life stage (i.e., care of young children or their own health problems). Studies of the effects of family caregiving have documented difficulties, including financial hardship, physical health problems, and, most pervasively, emotional and mental health concerns (Horowitz, 1985). Likewise, the economic implications of deferred work force participation may affect more than one family generation. Clearly, the impact of caregiving on relationships between generations and among all family members has implications for long-term care decision-making as is discussed by Sarah Brakman (Chap. 9), Nancy Jecker (Chap. 8), and John Arras (Chap. 10).

One major policy issue in long-term care concerns the role of the family in relation to the formal service system (Stone, 1991). With increasing fiscal constraints at federal, state, and local levels, families have been expected to respond to the demographic challenge of increasing numbers of disabled older people who require care for longer periods of time. As discussed in the next section, such support services as in-home respite care and day care and economic support to caregiving families have not expanded much. One of the principal concerns has been the "fear of substitution," that is, that expansion of publicly financed long-term care services would produce a substantial reduction in the activities of primary caregivers. In the few community care programs in which this issue has been systematically addressed, this fear has found no support. Family members have not drastically reduced their efforts on behalf of disabled elderly when formal services were provided (Christianson, 1988; Moscovice, Davidson, and McCaffrey, 1988). However, as explained in the section on demonstration studies, the failure to reduce overall public costs by providing home and community-based services has not allayed fears about the potential for reductions in family care. Future long-term care users are expected to have greater economic resources, but they are expected to have fewer available informal or family care resources because their families are smaller and more widespread.

*Financing and Organization of Formal Long-Term
Care Services*

Although families are the principal providers of long-term care, formal services–both institutional and noninstitutional—exist to meet some of the needs of persons who require this care. As outlined in Figure 2, the range of services includes care providers at home, in community settings, and in a growing variety of housing and institutional facilities. For most disabled Americans in most communities, however, such an ideal continuum of care exists only on paper. Across the country, availability of institutional as well as home- and community-based services varies considerably. Understanding this diversity and the often limited availability of help beyond the family requires some attention to the facts of long-term care policy and financing. In long-term care as in other aspects of U.S. health care delivery, "form follows funding" (Kane and Kane, 1990, p. 416). Because U.S. long-term care policy and financing are decentralized, categorical, and limited (Benjamin, 1992, p. 14), there is no long-term care system but a fragmented array of different programs and many gaps in what is needed, especially outside of institutions. The following facts regarding long-term care financing are key to comprehending the current nonsystem of care.

1. *Major differences and divisions exist between the financing of acute and long-term care for the elderly.* The inception of Medicare in 1965 established major divisions between these two types of care. Medicare provides insurance coverage primarily for acute care to virtually all persons aged 65 and older, regardless of income. The Medicare system underwrites a large portion of federal expenditures for home care, but its benefits are limited to skilled nursing, therapeutic services, durable medical equipment, and short-term care by home health aides, provided that the services are related to acute health conditions. Although Medicare provides coverage for short-term stays in skilled nursing facilities, total Medicare spending amounts to about 4 percent of nursing home expenditures. Unlike Medicare, the other public insurance program, Medicaid, reimburses recipients for nursing home care, and on a much more limited basis for home- and community-based care. Originally established as a federal-state medical insurance program for low-income persons, Medicaid has gradually shifted to become the primary public funding source for long-term care. The medical model of service,

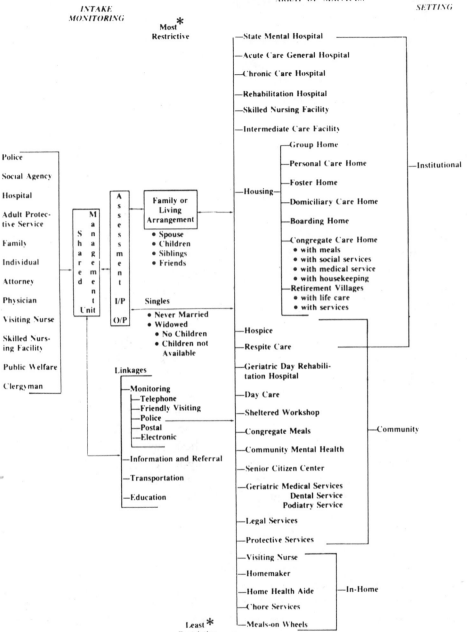

Figure 2. Inventory of recommended available services, appropriate to a long-term care/support system. *The classification of from most to least restrictive is a general view of services and may vary within each service. *Source:* Brody and Masciocchi (1980).

rather than the social service model, to which long-term care is more closely related, persists in the Medicaid regulations. Along with this medical heritage, long-term care has a "welfare heritage," as noted by Holstein and Cole (Chap. 2). Thus, despite the substantial cost of long-term care in a nursing home (an average of more than $37,000 a year), financial assistance is still provided only to individuals and families who qualify because of low income and some depletion of assets. Unlike the Medicare guidelines, which are uniform based on a single funding source, the partially state-financed Medicaid system allows variations in eligibility requirements, service plans, and payment levels across states. Medicaid is therefore a welfare, not an entitlement program.

The variability in state guidelines produces severe inequities in per capita expenditures, and it creates substantial problems for elders and families who cross state boundaries as they attempt to make long-term care plans. The inequities in quality and availability of care are especially large in community care, but they also persist in nursing home care. In obtaining long-term care, the experience of the three older families previously described would vary greatly, depending on their community and state of residence. In some states, for example, Medicaid funding might give Mrs. Weinbrach more hours of home care than in others. The adult day care being provided to Mrs. West is Medicaid-funded in some states, with varying eligibility, but in others it is a completely private cost. Should Mrs. James eventually require nursing home care and be eligible for Medicaid, she might not be able to locate a bed in states in which Medicaid reimbursement rates are far below those of Medicare and private insurances. As one example of the inequity among state programs, New York and California offer personal care services to more broadly defined recipient groups and consequently spent 56 percent of the estimated total federal public expenditures for home- and community-based services in 1992 (Administration on Aging, 1993). Most of these funds came from Medicaid.

Under Medicaid legislation states may provide some home health or personal care services through the Medicaid state plan or as part of the home- and community-based services waiver authority enacted by Congress in 1981 (Justice, 1990). Under the Medicaid Waiver Program, states may offer a range of home care services to a specified number of individuals who otherwise would require nursing home care financed by Medicaid. This has encouraged many states to develop an innovative array of services. But, the total number of individuals helped is small compared to the total population in need (Binstock, Post, and White-house, 1992).

2. *Individuals and families pay for a significant portion of long-term care.* As shown in Table 1, not all disabled elderly people use formal services. Most of those who use long-term care pay for it from their own or their family's income or assets until they qualify for Medicaid (Wiener, 1990; for elaboration of Medicaid eligibility, see Jecker, Chap. 8). Expenditures for nursing home care are paid in roughly equal shares by private individuals and government agencies. Government agencies pay for 48.5 percent of nursing home expenditures, primarily through Medicaid. Although public programs other than Medicaid provide some help to disabled elders, Leutz et al. (1992) showed that only one in eight disabled elders living in the community relies on a public payer of care and that the others depend on assistance that they can buy or their families can provide.

Until the 1980s Medicaid, personal financial resources, and, to a limited degree, Medicare were the only means of paying for nursing home care. Since then, private financing plans, particularly for private long-term care insurance, have been multiplying. The plans vary significantly. Coverage of nursing home care is the principal benefit, with most but not all policies including some coverage of home care. Many policies exclude custodial care needs (such as assistance with activities of daily living without a skilled need) and care for persons with Alzheimer's disease. Choice of coverage and the purchaser's age determine the policy price—the older the purchaser, the higher the price, of course. There are many divergent opinions regarding the market potential of long-term care insurance as well as how public policy should relate to this financing option (Leutz et al., 1992; Rivlin and Wiener, 1988). Even the most optimistic projections of the market (which range from 16 to 68 percent of persons 65 and older) acknowledge, however, that a large portion of Americans will not have private insurance coverage, including persons of any age who already need long-term care (Leutz et al., 1992; Pepper Commission, 1990). Currently only 4 to 5 percent of the elderly have any private long-term care insurance, and about 1 to 2 percent of total nursing home expenditures for the elderly are paid by private insurance (Vladeck, Miller and Clauser, 1993; Wiener and Hixon Illston, 1994).

3. *Federal and state funding, provided through multiple program categories, results in fragmentation of benefits for the separate but interrelated medical, social, and income needs of older people.* The scope of this chapter prohibits a detailed review of all current public financing mechanisms for long-term care. However, a brief listing of current sources reveals the challenge that confronts consumers of long-term care or the people who try to obtain services for them. In addition to Medicare and Medicaid, which have separate but overlapping missions and target populations, other public programs have a limited role in paying for one or more long-term care services. Programs available to some extent in most communities include Social Service Block Grant funds (Title XX of the Social Security Act), Title III of the Older Americans Act, and the Department of Veterans Affairs (DVA, formerly the Veterans' Administration), which provides some modest financial assistance for disabled veterans, primarily men. The DVA also either operates or provides some funding for other respite or home care programs.

Of federal Social Service Block Grant funds intended to enable states to provide a variety of services to children and adults, only some are for persons with chronic care needs (home-based services and day care in particular). Although they are not required to do so, states may target services to low-income individuals, and they may charge fees on a sliding scale. In some states Title XX funds are administered in coordination with Older Americans Act funds; in others these programs have separate bureaucracies, creating confusion and barriers to coordinating care for an individual client.

The U.S. Administration on Aging (AoA) channels funds to each state so that a network of Area Agencies on Aging can provide some of the nutrition, home care, home maintenance, transportation, access, and other services listed in Figure 2. AoA services are targeted to persons 60 years of age and older without explicit income or fee requirements.

Complementing these federal programs, which have their own entitlement and eligibility requirements, most states have one or more programs to fund some home- and community-based services. In 1992, state programs funded through general revenue accounted for 11 percent of the total public outlay for home- and community-based services. Many of these programs are administered through the aging network.

Older people with chronic health problems continue to require shelter and an adequate physical and social environment. Local voluntary agencies typically seek to meet needs that are not adequately fulfilled by public services and that exceed the ability to pay of most older people and their families. One outgrowth of the diversity of separate programs serving functionally impaired older people has been strong support for the development of case management as a strategy to coordinate service delivery for frail older people. Case management takes various shapes, which I shall discuss later.

4. *Public financing of long-term care has been heavily biased toward payment for institutional long-term care and medical needs and not for formal home and community care.* Even though public expenditures for community-based long-term care have increased more rapidly than for nursing home care over the past decade, the bias toward public reimbursement of nursing homes remains in place. Estimates for 1993 were that 71 percent of all publicly funded long-term care would be for institutional services, leaving only 29 percent for home- and community-based care (Vladeck, Miller, and Clauser, 1993). Moreover, despite the substantial public investment, concerns about the quality of nursing home care persist, along with the hardships some families face in finding a nursing home that will provide the care reimbursed by Medicaid. Providing public funds primarily for nursing home care clearly assumes that informal care providers will be the major source of assistance to most of the long-term care population in the community, thus reinforcing a long history (Holstein and Cole, Chap. 2).

Sources of Formal Care

The sources of formal long-term care include nursing homes, residential services, and home and community care; each will be discussed in turn.

Nursing Home Care

Given the dominance of funding for institutional care, it follows that nursing homes are the "bulwark of current long-term care provision" (Kane and Kane, 1987, p. 54). Although there is considerable variability among states with respect to occupancy rate, bed to population ratios, and other characteristics, nationwide the nursing home system is primarily involved in caring for people with significant disabilities and often medically complex needs who require both postacute and long-term care. Most nursing homes in the United States are proprietary businesses; slightly less than half are part of a national chain. As Holstein and Cole indicate (Chap. 2), nursing home care has always been a business as well as a mode of meeting long-term care needs. The desire to improve the quality of care has resulted in persistent attention to nursing home standards and regulations mandated by the federal government and implemented by the states. The wide gap in reimbursement by Medicaid and private payers has also brought along problems of access to nursing homes for persons who must depend on public financial support. Apart from periodic concerns with quality issues in nursing home life, the most troubling issue is fiscal policy. Because Medicaid is now the fastest growing expense of many states, there is great concern about how to respond to the needs of the growing older population without creating state fiscal crises (Somers, 1993; Leutz et al., 1992).

Other Residential Options

Nursing homes are the best known but not the only group residential option for older people with disabilities. Holstein and Cole (Chap. 2) discuss the longstanding role of board and care facilities or group quarters. As listed in Figure 2, a variety of residential facilities are available to older people who are unable or prefer not to maintain independent homes. Most states have both licensed and unlicensed forms of housing (called retirement homes, personal care homes, board and care facilities, etc.) with some services, and these settings are often designed for persons of different levels of income. Public subsidy is available in some states, for example, to people with low incomes who need adult foster care or similar housing. An option developed specifically for wealthier old people is the continuing care retirement community, also known as life care. Originally organized by old religious organizations, the continuing care retirement community (CCRC) combines housing, health care, and social supports for persons of at least middle income and generally retirement age (Somers, 1993). In 1992 approximately 250,000 older people were living in 700 CCRCs in forty states, with cost being prohibitive for many older people (Somers, 1993).

Concern for the cost and efficiency of delivering home care in separate dwellings and an interest in being more responsive to consumer preferences have produced growing attention to the concept of assisted living. In their recent study of this option, Rosalie Kane and Keren Wilson defined assisted living as "any group residential program other than a licensed nursing home that provides personal care for persons with impairments in performance of ADLs and has the capacity to meet unscheduled needs for assistance" (Kane and Wilson, 1993, p. 1). Examining a variety of settings that meet this definition, Kane and Wilson identified several environments that provide "individualized personal care in accommodations that offer more privacy, space and dignity, than are typically available in nursing home care, and at lower cost" (Kane and Wilson, 1993, p. vii). As they noted, the development of assisted living has been a private market phenomenon, and its cost-saving potential, while meeting the needs of disabled old people, is increasingly being examined by state governments. The variability of subsidized assisted living is considerable both within and across the fifty states.

Home and Community Care

The best known long-term care services delivered in the home or community address the elder's basic need for personal care. Information about private payment for services is limited, but data on collective public spending by service category are available. According to information from the AoA on federal and state expenditures in 1992, the services purchased most frequently with public dollars were personal care, homemaker chore service, and home health aide service (Administration on Aging, 1993). Other services generally supported by either federal or state dollars include home-delivered meals, respite care, adult day care or day health service, and transportation (Short and Leon, 1990). Although receiving care at home is the preference of most older people, the nature of current home care services may introduce many unwanted changes into their daily lives (Collopy, Dubler, and Zuckerman, 1990). As Wetle discusses in detail in Chapter 4, program regulations rather than consumers may determine what kind of help is provided, how, and by whom. Professionals and policy makers acknowledge several unresolved issues regarding how to promote the most effective relationship between families (the dominant care providers) and formal services and how to ensure the quality of services (Stone, 1991).

The Role of Case Management

Care or case management, which is both an administrative function and a service, has been an essential feature of nearly all community care programs and demonstration projects. Its principal function, as defined by White (1987), is to obtain essential resources for clients in collaboration with both formal and informal sources. The appeal of case management is reflected in its consistent inclusion in federal and state legislative proposals as well as its adoption by insurance carriers responsible for long-term care policies.

Although the terminology is often similar, case management has many different meanings and varies greatly among programs. Applebaum and Austin (1990) observed that case management is popular as a policy reform approach to long-term care because it fits into operating delivery systems and does not require restructuring of the interorganizational relationships. Unfortunately, this shifts the burden of many difficult decisions about allocation of resources to the case manager, as discussed by Kane and Wetle in their chapters. Applebaum and Austin (1990) distinguished case management models by the methods by which case managers implement a given client's plan of care. Three commonly identified models include the broker model, the service management model, and the managed care model. In the broker model, a case manager may identify needs and make referrals to implement a client's care plan but has no guarantee that the service will be delivered and little or no ability to spend service dollars on the client's behalf. In the service management model, the case manager has the authority to purchase services that are not beyond a predetermined financial cost cap. The managed care model resembles the service management model with respect to the case manager's authority to buy services for the clients, but the case management agency operates with prospective financing, that is, the agency is prepaid a specific amount for providing case management and other services. Typically, states with community care programs use some version of the service management model, generally restricting a care plan's cost cap to 60 to 80 percent of the cost of stay in a Medicaid reimbursed nursing home.

In addition to the client-specific goals of case management, broadly defined system goals focus on cost containment, quality, and efficiency in the delivery of long-term care. Although case management methods have become popular among policy makers concerned with cost containment, there is no evidence that this service can routinely reduce long-term care costs. As Terrie Wetle (Chap. 4) and Rosalie Kane (Chap. 5) report, case managers have multiple roles in the long-term care system, and they confront several dilemmas in trying to fulfill both client-centered as well as program-centered goals.

Research and Demonstration Lessons

During the past two decades, improvements in the financing and service provision of long-term care for the elderly have been studied in several research and demonstration projects. To the disappointment of advocates and consumers, the preponderance of research evidence showed that expansion of home and community services does not save public funds (Kemper, Applebaum, and Harringan, 1987; Weissert, Cready, and Pawelak, 1988). Community care interventions have increased health costs because they failed to reduce the use of institutions sufficiently to offset the increased demand for and use of community-based care. Although a given individual may be cared for at a lower cost in the community than in an institution, aggregate program costs are higher. The disappointing findings regarding cost are accompanied by limited improvements in health status and well-being. The most consistent improvements have been achieved in the area of client and caregiver satisfaction and in the reduction of unmet needs (Weissert, Cready, and Pawelak, 1988). Because old people and their families strongly prefer to live in the home and community, policy analysts and other professionals have continued to identify and pursue strategies to increase the cost effectiveness of publicly financed care. Among the strategies suggested are targeting services to *severely* disabled individuals, focusing on hospital diversion, linking supportive housing and services, and improving utilization control (Weissert, 1991; Vladeck, Miller, and Clauser, 1993).

Two demonstration projects are currently addressing a major theme in both financing and delivery of services to individuals with chronic care needs, namely, the integration of long-term and acute care. The two are the Program of All-inclusive Care for the Elderly (PACE demonstration and the PACE prototype, On Lok Senior Health Services) and the Social Health Maintenance Organization (S/HMO Demonstration). Although the models are different, both multisite demonstrations are exploring prepaid programs that combine comprehensive medical care coverage with community long-term care benefits for persons with Medicare and sometimes Medicaid as well (Vladeck, Miller, and Clauser, 1993).

Looking toward the Future

Given the myriad problems of access, supply, and quality of long-term care, it is not surprising that numerous proposals for financing reform have been made during the past several years, including the 1990 Pepper Commission report advocating universal coverage of long-term care, public-private partnerships using insurance models, and various revisions of Medicare and Medicaid that would integrate acute care and chronic care like the S/HMO and PACE projects.

President Clinton's proposal for long-term care currently before the 1994 Congress contains elements of several of these approaches by calling for expanded home care for severely disabled persons of all income groups, favorable tax clarification (treating long-term care benefits with tax-favored status), and further regulation of private insurance. However, many competing legislative proposals for health care reform eliminate any expansion of long-term care benefits, so that the fear about costs at a time of budget deficit and social welfare retrenchment may overwhelm the proposals to improve long-term care (Binstock and Murray, 1992). The issues of long-term care policy are complex, in part because they are intertwined with central issues in income transfer, health care policy, and housing policy (Congressional Budget Office, 1991). Joshua Wiener and Laurel Hixon Illston examined the three global policy issues to be addressed in any national long-term care policy: where long-term care fits in overall health care reform, the mix of public and private services, and the allocation of resources to institutional services versus home and community-based care. Wiener and Hixon Illston noted that architects of a new public program of long-term care must address the old and persistent questions: "What is the role of the states? How will expenditures be controlled? Will there be a broad benefit package and how does this affect entitlement to services? Will acute care and long-term care services be integrated? How will elderly and nonelderly disabled persons be cared for? And, finally, how will adequate financing be assured?" (p. 405).

Implications for Long-Term Care Decision Making

In this review, I have attempted to identify the significant social and economic constraints on long-term care born of the inequitable, nonsystem of care currently in place. We have no national policy on long-term care. Current public payment for long-term care emphasizes medical need and, therefore, medical values which may conflict with other psychosocial values and issues of personal meaning as discussed by Collopy (Chap. 7) and Agich (Chap. 6). Furthermore, societal expectations of family members do not reflect understanding of the diversity and changing nature of family relationships, the well-documented strains of caregiving, and the implications of an aging society. Old people confronting chronic illness, family members concerned with their well-being, and professionals in health and social services inherit the unresolved dilemmas created by this nonsystem and the absence of policy. The following chapters explore these dilemmas.

REFERENCES

Administration on Aging. (1993). *Profile of State Administered Home and Community Based Services for the Functionally Impaired Elderly.* Washington, D.C.: Administration on Aging.

Applebaum, R., and Austin, C. (1990). *Long-Term Care Case Management.* New York: Springer Publishing Co.

Benjamin, A.E. (1992). An overview of in-home health and supportive services for older persons. In M.G. Ory and A.P. Duncker (eds.), *In-Home Care for Older People: Health and Supportive Services.* Beverly Hills, Calif.: Sage Publications.

Binstock, R.H., and Murray, T.H. (1992) The politics of developing appropriate care for dementia. In R.H. Binstock, S.G. Post, and P.J. Whitehouse (eds.), *Dementia and Aging: Ethics, Values, and Policy Choices.* Baltimore: Johns Hopkins University Press.

Binstock, R.H., Post, S.G., and Whitehouse, P.J. (1992). The challenges of dementia. In R.H. Binstock, S.G. Post, and P.J. Whitehouse (eds.), *Dementia and Aging: Ethics, Values, and Policy Choices.* Baltimore: Johns Hopkins University Press.

Brody, E.M. (1985). Parent care as a normative family stress. *Gerontologist, 25*: 19–29.

Brody, E.M., and Brody S.J. (1989). The informal system of health care. In C. Eisdorfer, P.A. Kessler, and A.N. Spector (eds.), *Caring for the Elderly: Reshaping Public Policy,* pp. 259–277. Baltimore: Johns Hopkins University Press.

Brody, S.J. and Magel, J.S. (1984). DRG: The second revolution in health care for the elderly. *Journal of the American Geriatrics Society, 32*: 676–679.

Brody, S.J., and Magel, J.S. (1989). Long-term care: The long and short of it. In C. Eisdorfer, P.A. Kessler, and A.N. Spector (eds.), *Caring for the Elderly: Reshaping Public Policy,* pp. 235–258. Baltimore: Johns Hopkins University Press.

Brody, S.J., and Masciocchi, C. (1980). Data for long-term care planning by health systems agencies. *American Journal of Public Health, 70*: 1194–1198.

Christianson, J.B. (1988). The evaluation of the national long-term care demonstration: The effect of channeling on informal caregiving. *Health Services Research,* 23: 99–117.

Collopy, B., Dubler, N., and Zuckerman, C. (1990). The ethics of home care: Autonomy and accommodation. *Hastings Center Report,* (Special Supplement): 1–16.

Congressional Budget Office. (1991). *Policy Choices for Long-Term Care.* Washington, D.C.: U.S. Congress.

Estes, C.L., Swan, J.H., and Associates (1993). *The Long-Term Care Crisis, Elders Trapped in the No-Care Zone.* Beverly Hills, Calif.: Sage Publications.

George, L.K., and Maddox, G. (1989). Social and behavioral aspects of institutional care. In M. Ory and K. Bond (eds.), *Aging and Health Care: Social Science and Policy Perspectives,* pp. 116–141. London: Ruttledge.

Harrington, C., Newcomer, R.J., Estes, C.L., and Associates. (1985). *Long-Term Care of the Elderly.* Beverly Hills, Calif.: Sage Publications.

Hing, E. (1990). *Long-Term Care for the Functionally Dependent Elderly: Vital and Health Statistics, Series 13; Data from the National Health Interview: Survey No. 104.* Hyattsville, Md.: National Center for Health Statistics.

Horowitz, A. (1985). Family caregiving to the frail elderly. In C. Eisdorfer (ed.), *Annual Review of Gerontology and Geriatrics,* Vol. 5. New York: Springer Publishing Co.

Justice, D. (1990). State community-based care systems. *Generations,* 14(2): 45–49.

Kane, R.A., and Kane, R.I. (1987). *Long-Term Care: Principles, Programs and Policies.* New York: Springer Publishing Co.

Kane, R.L., and Kane, R.A. (1989). Transitions in long-term care. In M. Ory and K. Bond (eds.), *Aging and Health Care: Social Science and Policy Perspectives.* New York: Routledge.

Kane, R.L., and Kane, R.A. (1990). Healthcare for older people: Organizational and policy issues. In R.H. Binstock and L.K. George (eds.), *Handbook of Aging and the Social Sciences.* 3rd ed., pp. 415–437. San Diego: Academic Press.

Kane, R.A., and Wilson, K.B. (1993). *Assisted Living in the United States: A New Paradigm for Residential Care for Frail Older Persons?* Washington, D.C.: American Association of Retired Persons Public Policy Institute.

Kemper, P. (1992). The use of formal and informal home care by the disabled elderly. *Health Services Research,* 27: 421–451.

Kemper, P., Applebaum, R., and Harrigan, M. (1987). Community care demonstrations: What have we learned? *Health Care Financing Review,* 8: 87–100.

Kemper, P., and Murtaugh, C.M. (1991). Lifetime use of nursing home care. *New England Journal of Medicine,* 324: 595–600.

Kovar, M.G. (1988). Aging in the eighties, people living alone—two years later. In *Data from the 1984 and 1986 Longitudinal Study of Aging Interviews. Advance Data from Vital and Health Statistics,* no. 149. Hyattsville, Md.: National Center for Health Statistics.

Leutz, W.N., Capitman, J.A., MacAdam, M., and Abrahams, R. (1992). *Care for Frail Elders: Developing Community Solutions.* Westport, Conn.: Auburn House.

Liu, K., Manton, K.G., and Liu, B.M. (1985). Home care expenses for the disabled elderly. *Health Care Financing Review,* 7: 51–58.

Moscovice, I., Davidson, G., and McCaffrey, D. (1988). Substitution of formal and informal care for the community based elderly. *Medical Care,* 26: 971–981.

Oriol, W. (1993). Long-term care: Options for the future. *Issues in Aging.* Washington, D.C.: National Council on the Aging.

Ory, M.G., and Duncker, A.P. (eds.., (1992). *In-Home Care for Older People: Health and Supportive Services.* Beverly Hills, Calif.: Sage Publications.

Pepper Commission. (1990). *Access to Health Care and Long-Term Care for All Americans: Recommendations to the Congress.* Washington, D.C.: U.S. Bipartisan Commission on Comprehensive Health Care.

Rivlin, A.M., and Wiener, J.M. (1988). *Caring for the Disabled Elderly: Who Will Pay?* Washington, D.C.: Brookings Institution.

Rowland, D., and Lyons, B. (1991). The elderly population in need of home care. In D. Rowland and B. Lyons (eds.), *Financing Home Care: Improving Protection for Disabled Elderly People,* pp. 3–26. Baltimore: Johns Hopkins University Press.

Rowland, D., Lyons, B., Newman, P., Salangicoff, A., and Taghavi, L. (1988). *Defining the Functionally Impaired Elderly Population.* Washington, D.C.: Public Policy Institute.

Short, P.F., and Leon, J. (1990). *Use of Home and Community Services by Persons Ages 65 and Older with Functional Difficulties.* DHHS Publication no. (PHS) 90-3466, National Medical Expenditure Survey Research Findings, 5, Agency for Health Care Policy Research. Rockville, Md.: Public Health Service.

Somers, A.R. (1993). "Lifecare": A viable option for long-term care for the elder. *Journal of the American Geriatrics Society,* 41: 188–191.

Stone, R. (1991). Familial obligations: Issues for the nineties. *Generations,* 15: 47–50.

Stone, R., Cafferata, G., and Sangl, J. (1987). Caregivers of the frail elderly: A national profile. *Gerontologist, 27:* 616–626.

Stone, R.I., and Murtaugh, C.M. (1990). The elderly population with chronic functional disability: Implications for home care eligibility. *Gerontologist, 30:* 491–496.

Vladeck, B.C., Miller, N.A., and Clauser, S.B. (1993). The changing face of long-term care. *Health Care Financing Review, 14:* 5–23.

Weissert, W.G. (1991). A new policy agenda for home care. *Health Affairs, 10(2):* 67–77.

Weissert, W.G., Cready, C.M., and Pawelak, J.E. (1988). The past and future of home- and community-based long-term care. *Milbank Quarterly, 66:* 309–388.

White, M. (1987). Case management. In G. Maddox (ed.), *Encyclopedia of Aging,* pp. 92–96. New York: Springer Publishing Co.

Wiener, J.M. (1990). Which way for long-term-care financing? *Generations, 14:* 5–9.

Wiener, J.M., and Hixon Illston, L. (1994). Health care reform and long-term care. *Gerontologist, 34:* 402–408.

Yeo, G.W. (1993). Ethnicity and nursing homes: Factors affecting use and successful components for culturally sensitive care. In C. Barresi and D.E. Stull (eds.), *Ethnic Elderly and Long-Term Care,* pp. 161–177. New York: Springer Publishing Co.

II PRACTICE CONSIDERATIONS

CHAPTER FOUR

Ethical Issues and Value Conflicts Facing Case Managers of Frail Elderly People Living at Home

Terrie Wetle

Case management is increasingly important in the lives of frail older persons. Federal, state, and private initiatives intended to improve access to community-based services, as well as control costs through targeted eligibility assessment and tighter gatekeeping, have increased the demand for case management services and broadened the roles of case managers (Applebaum and Austin, 1990). These new demands have begun to focus attention on the ethical issues and value conflicts that arise for case managers, their agencies, and the clients they serve (Kane and Caplan, 1993; Kane, 1988a).

The purpose of this chapter is to provide an overview of these ethical issues and value conflicts and to discuss their implications for both the practice of case management and client autonomy. In the first section I present a taxonomy of ethical issues that exist in the relationships of case managers and their clients, case managers and families, case managers and health care providers, as well as issues that arise within and among agencies. Next, I examine limits in the delivery system and the associated ethical implications for autonomy of case-managed older persons who live in the community. In the third section, which presents a series of contradictions in case management, I examine differences between client-centered theory and directive practice. The concluding section is a discussion of perceptions of client autonomy in case-managed care, including a review of the literature on concordance between providers and patients, and findings from a recent study on autonomy in

The work on which this chapter is based was supported by the Retirement Research Foundation.

case management. Case-managed clients' perceptions are compared with those of their case managers with regard to major elements of autonomy, including information-sharing, participation in decision making, and level of client choice.

A Taxonomy of Ethical Issues in Case Management

It can be argued that frail elderly case management clients are at ethical risk, meaning at risk of being excluded from decisions regarding their care, at risk of not receiving the least restrictive, most appropriate care, and at risk in social policy decisions (Wetle, 1987). This argument is based on anecdotal observations as well as research data that show advanced age to be associated with less than optimal treatment for breast and other cancers (Greenfield et al., 1987), exclusion from health care decisions (Wetle et al., 1988), exclusion from care plan decisions (MaloneBeach, Zarit, and Spore, 1992; Simon-Rusinowitz and Hofland, 1993; Clemens et al., 1994), and a greater likelihood of nursing home placement (Fox, 1981). Whether all these differences in treatment are due to ageism or other factors remains to be determined. Certainly, advanced age carries increased risk of physical frailty as well as cognitive impairment and increased dependence, factors that have each been shown to influence care decisions.

Larger societal issues seem also to influence these individual health care decisions. The "old-old" are the fastest growing segment of our population. As health care costs spiral upward for people of all ages, it is not surprising that policy makers have recently focused primary attention on controlling the costs of care for older Americans. The combination of demographic trends, dramatic increases in public spending during a period of budget constraints, and societal and professional ageism place frail old clients at special risk.

Case management (or care coordination) involves an array of functions that may vary among practice settings. The basic functions include outreach (case finding), assessment (usually structured, comprehensive, and multidimensional), development and implementation of a care plan, monitoring of service delivery (quality of care), and reassessment of clients (Kane and Thomas, 1993). Practitioners also generally agree that their functions include client advocacy, determination of eligibility for a variety of public programs or private insurance benefits (gatekeeping), record-keeping, negotiation with family members and other providers of care, and observation of a variety of federal, state, and agency rules and regulations. The work is conducted in an environment of increasing competition, shrinking budgets, and rising demands.

Ethical Issues Concerning Clients

Societal and professional issues that influence case management practice include concepts of nonmaleficence, beneficence, paternalism, perceptions of the client's best interests, and justice. Perceptions of family values and obligations also play a role. Case managers frequently find themselves engaging in "values calculus" as they identify and weigh competing and complementary values in case management decisions. The relevant concepts, described briefly (see also Beauchamp and Childress, 1994), are the following.

Nonmaleficence, the strong proscription of doing harm to others, is supported by societal values, professional ethics, and criminal and civil law. Expressed by the phrase "first, do no harm," this principle is found in the professional ethical codes of both nursing and social work, the disciplines of most professional case managers. The American Nurses Association (ANA) Code for Nurses (1976) states, for example, that "the nurse's primary commitment is to the client's care and safety" (Section 3.1).

Beneficence, simply put, is doing good for others, or generally promoting their welfare. As the basis of case management practice, beneficence is embodied in the ethical codes of nursing and social work. The National Association of Social Workers (NASW) Code of Ethics (1990) pledges social workers to promote "client best interest." The concept of "best interest" is closely tied to beneficence and refers to balancing the benefits and costs or risks of specific actions to determine the action most likely to benefit (or least likely to harm) the client.

Paternalism is the making of decisions for another. Two forms of paternalism are described; "weak" paternalism is making decisions for others who are unable to decide for themselves and is morally justified by principles of beneficence and justice. "Strong" paternalism refers to making decisions for others who are capable of doing so for themselves. Case managers frequently engage in "weak" paternalism for clients whose decision-making capacity is impaired, but the risk of "strong" paternalism is ever present.

One aspect of *justice* is the aggregate, fair distribution of benefits and harms among individuals. Although the case manager's role involves advocacy for specific clients, individual case managers and the agencies in which they work are also responsible for *populations* of clients. It is not uncommon for a single client's interests to be weighed against those of another client or group of clients.

Filial piety / family obligations are also considered in case management practice, although there is some disagreement about what these obligations entail for family members who provide care. The general cultural agreement, supported by common law, is that families do have special rights and responsibilities in health care decisions. At times, however, when the family disagrees, the case manager's role as client advocate may be to support a client's preference or choice.

Autonomy, a central value in Western thought, refers to the right of individuals to make decisions for themselves, free of coercion and undue influence. Autonomy has been conceptually divided into "agency" (the freedom to choose among options) and "action" (the freedom to carry out the chosen course of action) (Gadow, 1980). Case managers are able to enhance agency autonomy by providing information regarding eligibility, service alternatives, and individual client rights. They may enhance their clients' action autonomy by enabling them to act on decisions.

Much of case management involves balancing client autonomy with competing and complementary values and principles in care planning. The heterogeneity of preferences among frail elderly persons concerning their participation in care decisions, involvement of family members in decisions, and the nature of services they receive has been well documented. Case management clients may have physical conditions that limit their choices, cognitive or mental impairments that influence their judgment, and educational and social experiences that may constrain their expression of preferences. Clients' ethnicity, education, and cultural and personal experiences may influence their interest and willingness to participate in case management planning and decisions or even to express preferences. Individuals who have had a lifetime of negative experiences with authority figures, such as government workers or health professionals, may be reluctant to disagree or assert their wishes with case managers. Cultural differences in the timing or style of expressing preferences or providing information (Schensul, Torres, and Wetle, 1992) are differences that may lead the case manager to underestimate the importance of such expressions. Physical limitations and severity of illness not only limit the client's range of choices by dictating certain requirements of the physical environment, but they may, in the extreme, necessitate an unreasonably intensive or expensive care plan. Cognitive impairments affect the capacity to understand and to process information, as well as the ability to make judgments. Case managers are client advocates on the one hand; on the other they are charged with making decisions for persons who cannot decide for themselves.

Some caregivers tend to attribute cognitive impairment to very old persons or to other specific populations of older persons (Levkoff and Wetle, 1989; Iris, 1988), a legacy of the history described by Martha Holstein and Thomas Cole in Chapter 2. Questions of client competence are most likely to arise when the client makes choices that contradict the expectations or recommendations of case managers or family members and are therefore judged to be unreasonable. Determining the capacity to make decisions is an inexact science. "Competence" is a legal term, and although some cognitively impaired clients are formally determined to be "incompetent" by a probate court, most clients do not undergo this formal procedure. Most ethicists and clinicians prefer the concept of task-specific competence (Brody, 1993), recognizing that individuals may have the decisional capacity to make some decisions but not others. Formal assessment of competence or decisional capacity is complex and laden with ethical implications. Most case managers are not formally trained to perform comprehensive cognitive assessments nor to determine decisional capacity. In general, they report determining the decisional capacity of clients by "getting to know them" and by the quality of the clients' decisions. Special problems arise when clients are "eccentric," particularly those whose behavior brings them to public attention (Brody, 1993). The distinction between poor judgment as a result of cognitive impairment and unusual "life style" is not easy, and case managers sometimes play the role of "agents of community control," using "intrusive beneficence" to intervene with clients the community may find indecorous or otherwise troublesome (Collopy, 1993).

Nonetheless, case managers do make informal determinations of the competence of clients to participate in the care-planning process, and, in working with clients whose decision-making ability is considered to be impaired, use alternative strategies to implement care plans believed to be in the clients' best interest. It is not unusual, however, for case managers to go to extraordinary lengths for some cognitively impaired clients to determine their preferences and to develop care plans to help them remain at home even at substantial risk (Wetle et al., 1991). The level of effort case managers exert to enhance their cognitively impaired clients' autonomy varies among case managers, their agencies, and their clients (Clemens et al., 1994).

Although individual autonomy is a primary concern of competent clients, the application of traditional views of autonomy to home-care clients may have certain limitations. It can be argued that the privacy and familiar surroundings of one's home enhance decision making and the assertion of preferences. We must question, however, whether traditional concepts of autonomy are adequate and appropriate. George Agich (1990) argues that the abstract liberal concept of autonomy of rational individuals making independent choices is appropriate for the legal and political spheres, but not the moral one. He believes that a fuller concept is required, one that acknowledges the "social nature of human development and recognizes dependence as a non-accidental feature of the human condition" (Agich, 1990, p. 12). Such a view requires attention to individuals' history and development, including their experience of daily life. It also focuses on the communicative interactions between individuals, rather than on the current emphasis which makes informed consent an event rather than a process (Lidz, Applebaum, and Meisel, 1988). In the concept Agich develops later in this volume (Chap. 6), the case manager plays a major role in facilitating interstitial autonomy— that is, independence in performing everyday tasks for oneself—in developing the details of the client's care plan. And the case management client, because of the very conditions that make case management services appropriate, may be more likely to depend on relationships with family, neighbors, service providers, and others. The case manager may, therefore, be involved in helping the elder to negotiate spousal responsibility (Jecker, Chap. 8) and filial obligations (Brakman, Chap. 9) with careful attention to the subtle constraints of self-interest on those obligations (Arras, Chap. 10).

Ethical Issues Concerning Family Members

Care of frail older persons frequently involves family members and other informal care providers, which raises a variety of ethical concerns. The first question of ethical relevance is "Who is the client?" Although the family unit must be considered in care planning, the recognization that the interests of individual family members may conflict is critical. The desire of an elder hospitalized client to be discharged to her daughter's home may, for example, conflict with the daughter's or her husband's preferences and interests. Changing dependency relationships also may call into question formerly accepted family relationships and "ways of doing family business." Because we have no clear cultural expectations of what one generation is reasonably expected to do for another (Brakman, Chap. 9), feelings of guilt or abandonment may disturb already burdened relationships. Confusion regarding intergenerational expectations exists at both the public and the family level (Holstein and Cole, Chap. 2; Wilson, Chap. 3), causing resentment and anger, and may complicate care planning that involves integration of formal and informal supports.

The actual involvement of family members in care decisions raises several questions. First, the case manager must determine whom to involve as the most appropriate family members. Certainly, the competent client should be asked for permission to bring other family members into the discussion and to say who these family members are to be. If family members are part of the care plan, they must, of course, be involved in the planning process (Dubler, 1988).

Once the appropriate family member or members have been identified and the care questions clarified, the case manager provides additional assistance in the decision process. Two important guidelines for decision making are the concepts of substituted judgment and best interests of the client. The courts have increasingly encouraged the use of the substituted judgment standard, by which the family member determines what the incompetent client would want under these circumstances, if he or she were competent and able to express a preference. The decision maker is asked to think back to the relative's expressed wishes, actions, or other behaviors that would provide evidence of preferences. This is contrasted with best interest, under which decision makers determine what, in their opinion, is best for the client. Generally, the substituted judgment standard takes precedence, but if client preference is not known, then the best interest standard is used. Case managers sometimes face a difficult situation in which the family members' judgment in making decisions for a frail elder is shadowed by unresolved conflicts. The values inventory or values history discussed by Rosalie Kane in the next chapter can be a valuable aid in this process.

Ethical Issues among Professional Disciplines

Since the care of frail clients often requires a multidisciplinary approach that involves several different health care professionals, effective communication between case managers and the other health care professionals is critical to the success of case management. A review of the social work, nursing, and medical literature reveals little research concerning interaction of physicians and case managers, yet their relationship is often perceived as relatively ineffective and inefficient (Kapp, 1987; Feltes et al., 1994). Working relationships among case managers, physicians, and other health care providers reflect differences in professional training and the social environment in which they work (Mizrahi and Abramson, 1985; Huntington, 1981). The majority of case managers have backgrounds in either social work or nursing, both of which emphasize a holistic view of the patient or client in a broad social context. The training of physicians, in contrast, has always emphasized the biology of disease and episodic care of the patient (Makadon, 1985).

Value conflicts often arise among different types of professionals, or even similar professionals practicing in different agencies. For example, case managers in free-standing case management agencies reported higher thresholds of risk (they will "live with" higher levels of risk of injury or other harm to support a client's wish to stay at home) than might be customary for a home nursing agency care provider who is constrained by regulations or agency rules to provide a "twenty-four-hour" care plan (Wetle et al., 1991). This perception of a willingness to "go out on a limb" to support client autonomy is a frequent theme of case managers, who report feeling at odds with other professionals or agencies (and see themselves at risk of professional embarrassment or legal liability) as they advocate for clients (Clemens et al., 1994).

Members of different professions also have different informal codes of behavior that involve sharing of information about clients, communication among professionals, or styles of behavior. This is in part due to professional socialization and may also involve a form of professional chauvinism (i.e., my profession knows best what this client needs) (Feltes et al., 1994). The tension is exacerbated by disparate perspectives on teamwork that stem from different histories, values, and socialization processes (Mullaly, 1988). Social workers are taught the value of cooperation, while physicians are trained to take charge and assume leadership roles in multidisciplinary settings (Makadon, 1985). This is amplified by a strong medical social work tradition in which the superior status of physicians is acknowledged as a condition of social work's survival in medical organizations (Kerson, 1980; Kane, 1988a). These factors seem to create friction and hinder the development of a complementary interprofessional model. Tension derived from differential socialization and a lack of shared values, added to power and status differences among the professions, may actually undermine collaboration (Huntington, 1981; Kapp, 1987; Abramson and Mizrahi, 1987).

Ethical Issues for Case Managers and Agencies

As most case managers work for an agency or other formal organization, their personal and professional ethics and values may come into conflict with agency rules or constraints. Role conflicts, for example, that arise from competing demands are a frequent source of ethical concern. The case manager is at once required to be a client advocate, a gatekeeper in determining eligibility, and a cost saver. At times the best interests of a client may conflict with agency survival: when reimbursement is scarce, for example, or expenditures are capped, and the client requires a costly care plan. Conflicts between the desire to provide direct service and the demands of paperwork and administrative responsibilities often trouble case managers. Expanding case loads may diminish the intensity and quality of care planning and monitoring they provide to individual clients. Finally, case managers may feel that "ethical" expertise and backup support are lacking as they negotiate care plans for difficult clients and balance the safety and well-being of frail ones (Collopy, Chap. 7) against the clients' expressed desire to remain at home. The development of "ethical agencies," with administrators aware of these conflicts who would provide backup support through ethics committees and other resources, would help front line staff members to address these difficult issues. Some case managers report a sense of isolation or "loneliness," despite working in large, busy agencies. They attribute this to a feeling of being on the front line, making decisions for clients without sufficient backup or support (Clemens et al., 1994).

Kane, Penrod, and Kivnick (1993), reporting on the wide variation in staffing and experience among case management agencies, found these variations to influence understanding and ability to address role conflicts and other factors that may limit client autonomy. Even more significant, variations in the education, quality, and availability of workers to provide home-based services make a significant difference in the quality of life and respect for autonomy of clients. Much home-based care is provided by "unskilled" workers, usually women, who are paid the minimum wage to perform difficult and sometimes unpleasant tasks. Severe limitations in the availability of home care workers is a major problem for case managers in certain labor markets and limits their clients' options in care plans. Not uncommonly, home care workers differ from clients in ethnicity, cultural values, education, social class, preferred language, and life experience. Clients may make unacceptable demands, such as refusing the services of a worker whose race or ethnic background displeases them (Williams, 1993). A case manager's personal values, as well as such external factors as agency rules and diversity of the available worker pool, may prevent such a client's preferences from being met.

Ethical Issues for Agencies

Serving frail clients in an increasingly competitive environment, agencies may encounter value conflicts as a result of dumping unattractive clients (those difficult to serve, nonreimbursed, or reimbursed at low levels), turf battles (struggles over specific clients, populations of clients, or geographic catchment areas), and lack of coordination among multiple agencies serving specific clients. Successful case managers are sophisticated about the environment in which they work, including being savvy about local relationships among the competing agencies that serve their clients. Client advocacy requires scrutiny of these agencies' competitive behaviors, particularly those of the case manager's home agency, and an awareness that actions in the best interests of the agency may not necessarily coincide with those of the individual client.

Case management agencies and other direct service providers may have drastically different goals. While the case manager may emphasize client advocacy and respect for client autonomy, for example, visiting nurses may see the client's safety as more important. State Medicaid programs may focus on delivery of care in the least costly setting, while case managers may work to develop care plans more in keeping with the client's preferences, even at the loss of some efficiency. The differences may lead to misunderstandings and conflict over client care plans or agency practices.

Payment sources and reimbursement mechanisms for the case manager's services and other services in the care plan may constrain what case managers can do for their clients. Publicly funded services are limited by eligibility criteria, spending caps, and restrictions on types of services or providers or both. Moreover, many service agencies have "minimal units of service" (for example, a minimum home visit of four hours) that limit flexibility in care planning and may inflate the daily costs of care. Case managers who receive private payment directly from family members report feeling additionally constrained in advocating for the client when the family disputes the client's choices or preferences. Capitated payment mechanisms that cover populations of clients may pit one client's interests and preferences against those of another client or client group.

State regulatory criteria for certifying case management agencies (in states that certify or license case management agencies) may limit client choice, as may certain private health plans such as HMOs or long-term care insurers that may employ or contract with specific case managers or case management agencies. Other laws and regulations, such as the elder abuse reporting laws, require formal reports from case managers of suspected abuse or neglect even if the competent client chooses to stay in the "abusing" or "neglectful" situation.

Delivery System Limits: Ethical Implications for Case Management
Ethical Conflicts in the Service System

Case managers help clients obtain a complex array of services for acute, chronic, and home-based needs, from which they tailor flexible service packages into an individualized care plan. They advocate for and empower clients as they strive to ensure a safe environment, while helping the clients maintain independence as long as possible (Fanale et al., 1991; Moxley, 1989; Weil et al., 1985). Case managers provide care in a service and financing context much broader than the local environment. Biases in current public financing of long-term care restrict the autonomy of frail clients and the ability of case managers to develop optimal plans of care in the least restrictive environments. Reimbursement caps and eligibility restrictions for community and in-home services may result in unnecessary or premature institutional placement, just as pressures of the hospital prospective payment system may result in early discharge to less than optimal service settings.

Ageism in the service system affects both microlevel decisions concerning individual clients (such as whether or not to provide or withhold a specific treatment) and macrolevel decisions for a group or population (such as age limits for specific services). Explicit and implicit rationing of services is one way in which societal values may be expressed (Callahan, 1987). Although whether or not services will be rationed is the topic of current discussion, it must be acknowledged that services are already rationed according to several criteria (Wetle, 1991). Strategies for rationing are based on (*a*) ability to pay; (*b*) need; (*c*) entitlement; (*d*) first-come, first-served; (*e*) assessment of moral, social, or religious worth; (*f*) public or media pressure; (*g*) desirability as a research subject; (*h*) attractiveness as a client; and (*i*) risk of legal or financial liability (Churchill, 1988). Obviously, these rationing strategies frequently lead to inequities among clients and to social injustice.

Boundaries on Client Autonomy

The boundaries on autonomy raise concerns because of the particularly high value placed on this ethical principle. First, the fundamental assumption is that all persons are moral agents responsible for their own choices. Second, individuals are believed to be their own best judge of their own best interests, because those interests depend upon individual values and preferences (Tauer, 1993).

Competing demands complicate the case managers' struggle to address their clients' needs with ever-dwindling resources; they find themselves caught between "imperative duties" and "impossible demands" (Callahan, 1987). The dilemma is fueled by a lack of reimbursement for necessary services, fiscally driven access and discharge problems, and staff shortages that affect quality of care (Collopy, Dubler, and Zuckerman, 1990), as discussed earlier in this chapter. The recent shift in emphasis to cost containment and resource allocation gives rise to conflict between the tasks of gatekeeping and preserving client autonomy (Wetle et al., 1991; Clemens et al., 1994). Clients also exhibit substantial heterogeneity in their interest in and capacity for decision making, behavioral styles, coping mechanisms, social supports, values, and desired interventions. Disagreements between case managers and clients may raise ethical conflicts surrounding limitations of autonomy of elderly clients (Hennessy, 1989; Clemens et al., 1994).

The professional duty of beneficence may, at times, compete with support for client autonomy. The two professional disciplines most likely to be involved in case management, social workers and nurses, hold client self-determination as an important value in their professional codes of conduct. As Section 1.1 of the ANA Code for Nurses states,

> Whenever possible, clients should be fully involved in the planning and implementation of their own health care. Each client has the moral right to determine what will be done with his/her person; to be given the information

necessary for making informed judgments; to be told the possible effects of care and to accept, refuse, or terminate treatment. (ANA, 1976)

Principle II of the National Association of Social Workers Code of Ethics states

> ... the social worker's primary responsibility is to clients ... [to] maximize client self-determination. ... The social worker should provide clients with accurate and complete information regarding the extent and nature of services available to them ... apprise clients of the risks, rights, opportunities, and obligations associated with social services to them. (NASW, 1990)

The professional commitment to autonomy, however, often conflicts with the provider's duty of beneficence. The NASW Code of Ethics pledges social workers to "safeguard the interests and rights of clients" and to promote "client best interest" when acting on their behalf (NASW, 1990). The Code for Nurses states that nurses "should participate in ... activities ... which serve to safeguard clients" (ANA, 1988).

Bart Collopy (1993) discussed "intrusive beneficence," by which clients may be denied autonomy in the name of their own well-being as defined by others. He cautioned that social aberrations may thus be misconstrued as mental aberrations, physical frailty as cognitive frailty, and periodic lapses in function as proof of permanent incapacity (Katz, 1984; McCullough, 1984). Collopy also raised questions about beneficence as a means of community control.

Client self-determination is increasingly balanced against pressures from family members and care providers to ensure the client's safety and against professional and legal responsibility to promote the client's well-being and protection from harm (Austin et al., 1985; Hennessy, 1989; Kane, 1988b; Leutz et al., 1985). Even when case managers adopt a deliberately paternalistic approach to remove or reduce risks, the strategy should be to protect autonomy as much as possible by implementing the least restrictive and least intensive care plan options (Hennessy, 1989).

Public policy and practice ideals may also come into conflict. Fragmentation and gaps in the current system of care raise value conflicts as case managers struggle to accede to the wishes of the frail clients to remain at home but are unable to negotiate an adequate plan of care. Practice ideals and public policy may be in direct conflict as state and federal agencies implement new constraints in efforts to cut costs and balance budgets. Agencies are increasingly faced with balancing the needs of people currently served against the even greater needs for service of people in the community. In many states, clients are not eligible for some community-based public benefits, such as those under certain Medicaid waiver programs, unless they apply to a nursing home despite their expressed wish to remain at home. Long waiting lists for desirable facilities may also motivate case managers to urge their clients to apply for admission to a nursing home.

Contradictions in Case Management: Client-Centered Theory and Directive Practice

The ethical conflicts and limits of the delivery system have significant implications for the practice of case management. Our recent study (Clemens et al., 1994) that involved in-depth interviews with social work and nurse case managers revealed differences between client-centered philosophy and directive practice. We noted several types of theory/practice contradictions, including (*a*) client wishes versus system constraints; (*b*) the paradox of working to keep the client home versus the perceived inevitability of nursing home placement; (*c*) client-centeredness versus the case manager's care plan; (*d*) client self-determination versus strategies of persuasion; (*e*) consistent versus variable approaches to clients; and (*f*) informed consent in case management versus the realities of practice.

Client wishes versus system constraints. Nancy Wilson describes public policy and system constraints in Chapter 3. These include eligibility criteria for specific public programs, client-specific or agency-based caps on spending, oversight by protective services, family concerns and demands, and concerns for client safety. Case managers view state- and Medicaid-imposed cost caps as major limits on services. To some degree, these constraints dictate the comprehensiveness of the care plan, the nature of services provided, and the ability of the client to remain at home.

The placement paradox. Although keeping frail elderly clients at home is a primary goal of most case managers, many view nursing home placement as inevitable for most clients. Thus, while working to keep clients at home, case managers often simultaneously plan the clients' nursing home placement, and they sometimes develop strategies to overcome the clients' resistance. This leads to what has been called "the dance of placement."

Client-centeredness versus the case manager's safe plan of care. The central tool of case management, the care plan, is developed or negotiated by case managers and clients. Some case managers develop care plans more independently, however, based on their own assessment of the client's needs and best interests. The case manager's concerns for client safety are often used as justification for acting against the client's expressed wishes regarding care. Safety concerns are a frequent rationale for developing care plans "independent" of competent client input. Collopy (Chap. 7) cautions against treating independence and safety as a dichotomy.

Client self-determination versus strategies of persuasion. The goal of maintaining the client's autonomy must be reconciled with the client's potential need for nursing home care and for what may be perceived as intrusive services provided in the client's home. Case managers have several strategies, ranging from gentle persuasion to outright coercion, for achieving a frail but competent client's acceptance of a care plan. Again, the usual "trump card" in overriding autonomy is the concern for client safety.

Consistent versus variable approaches to clients. The value of consistency in care planning is sometimes contrasted with individualized approaches to specific clients; a willingness to "do more" may be based on client characteristics and the nature of the client–case manager relationship. Although support of client autonomy certainly leads to individualized approaches, the differences also include the degree to which case managers observe the autonomous wishes of clients, based on the clients' personal characteristics and unrelated to competence.

Informing the client about case management versus the reality of practice. Case managers typically emphasize their role as advisor in their initial contacts with clients, and they tell clients that they (clients) may terminate the case management "contract" at any time. However, case managers recognize a broader set of responsibilities that arise from regulatory and legal constraints; these are potential interventions they are less likely to share with clients. Full application of the doctrine of informed consent would mean that clients are informed of the various "risks" of accepting case management services, including the risk of institutional placement if the case manager determines that the client is no longer safe at home and can convince a probate court of that fact.

Perceptions of Client Autonomy in Case-Managed Care: Case Managers and Clients

Case managers seek to respond to their clients' needs and wishes (Moxley and Buzas, 1989) and to involve clients and their families in the planning and decision-making process. Thus, concordance between clients and case managers is crucial because it affects the clients' preferences for service and their perceptions of the way the service is rendered. These preferences and perceptions are related to a large array of other issues, including the client's desire to remain at home, the amount of information provided and the client's desire to be involved in decision-making, the client's health and need for services, the level of disagreement between client and case manager, the client–case manager working relationship, and the client's self-perception and level of self-determination.

Studies of concordance of the perceptions of clients and their professional caregivers have been limited, and, for the most part, they have not examined case management. Agreement between patients and health professionals has been studied primarily from a medical perspective (Davitz, 1969; Camp, 1988; Lynn-McHale and Belinger, 1988; Wetle, Cwikel, and Levkoff, 1988; Biggs, 1990). In a study of nursing home residents and their primary nurses, my colleagues and I (Wetle et al., 1988) observed disturbingly low concordance between the perceptions of nursing home residents and those of nurse caregivers regarding participation in medical decisions. The nurses were much more likely (63.8 percent) than the residents (28.3 percent) to believe that the residents were told all there was to know about their health care. The nurses also overestimated the residents' perceptions of the adequacy of information they received and their involvement in decision making. Compared to the residents' perceptions, nurses significantly underestimated their own level of participation in treatment decisions. Clemens (in press, 1994), in a study of discharge planning, also found a low level of congruence between the perceptions of the discharge planner and the family caregiver of participation in the discharge-planning process.

Perception of choice may also vary between patients and health care professionals. Rodin (1986) showed that the perception of control may be critical in old people's health and well-being. Studies of institutionalized elderly have demonstrated that an increased sense of control through choice affects health and longevity positively (Langer, 1983; Avorn and Langer, 1982; Kautzer, 1988). Hennessy (1989) found that the accumulation of restrictions on mundane aspects of daily living may diminish the elderly individual's quality of life. With regard to community-based care, MaloneBeach, Zarit, and Spore (1992) studied the caregivers of demented elderly people receiving case management and community-based services and found that the caregivers wanted to have more control over scheduling and the way services were delivered; they wanted to arrange for services directly and to participate in developing care plans. They also expressed a need to understand how and why case management decisions are made.

The observed lack of congruence between older patients' perceptions of their health circumstances and the perceptions of family members who play key roles in health care decisions complicates the case management task (Newquist, Hickey, and Rakowski, 1980). In one study (Rakowski and Hickey, 1979), patients and families tended not to agree about the older person's current health status, the patient's chief complaints and their cause, the expected length of treatment, and the treatment outcome. This central feature of long-term care decision making, "competing realities," is addressed in Chapter 11 of this volume by Laurence McCullough and coauthors.

Empirical studies of concordance in case management are few, but one such study sheds light on issues of concern. When my colleagues and I (Wetle et al., 1992) interviewed elderly case management clients and their case managers in matched interviews to identify the clients' preferences and perceptions, we found these to be related to information sharing, participation in making decisions, levels of disagreement, and level of client choice in the case management process.

Sharing information. We found that case managers estimated that they gave their clients more information about ways in which they could be helped than clients reported they received. These findings were similar to those of studies of other groups, such as nursing home residents and their nurse caregivers (Wetle et al., 1988) and hospitalized old people. Perhaps case managers overestimate their clients' level of understanding; they may not communicate as effectively as they believe they do, or they do not provide the information clients consider relevant. Case managers may provide information and choices their elderly clients do not remember, understand, or value.

Participation in decision making. The clients we interviewed (Wetle et al., 1992) saw themselves less involved in decision making than did their case managers, and they were less likely to report that case managers encouraged them to make their own decisions. Few studies have been conducted on levels of involvement of elders in health care decisions (Wetle, 1991), but several research groups have observed that elderly individuals wish to be involved and do actively participate when given the opportunity (Coulton et al., 1982; Lo, Saika, and Strull, 1985; Lo, McLeod, and Saika, 1986; Strull, Lo, and Charles, 1984). Case managers may be too indirect in their support of client decision making, or they may encourage decisions in areas of little importance to old clients. In the qualitative phase of the study by Clemens et al. (1994), we observed that case managers asked clients for their preferences concerning a major decision (the clients' desire to stay at home) but then made subsequent decisions for the clients in carrying out that wish. The clients' feelings of uninvolvement in decision making is underscored by Rosalie Kane and Authur Caplan's (1990) findings that nursing home residents place substantial importance on the "smaller" everyday decisions, such as when to bathe, what to wear, and when to make telephone calls. In Agich's terms (Chap. 6), interstitial or everyday autonomy is a significant dimension of the autonomy of elders in long-term care decision making.

Levels of disagreement. Case managers report more disagreements with clients than clients do. Because case managers recognize the clients' right to autonomy and self-determination, they may be more sensitive to disagreement. They may also be reluctant to reveal their disagreement to the client unless there is potential harm to the client or conflict with the needs of others. Alternatively, case managers may avoid direct confrontation with clients and use more subtle forms of persuasion or coercion to bring about desired outcomes. The elders may be fearful of open disagreement with someone they perceive as having power or control over them. Perhaps clients forget past disagreements with case managers once services are in place and they are satisfied. If clients are, indeed, not admitting or not openly discussing disagreements, encouraging such expression and providing a forum for voicing and resolving disagreements may be useful. An example of this is the preventive ethics approach to long-term care decision making described by McCullough and coauthors in Chapter 11 of this volume.

Level of client choice. When discussing the self-determination of clients, especially concerning services, the case managers perceived clients as having more choice than the clients reported. Similarly, MaloneBeach, Zarit, and Spore (1992) found that caregivers of demented case management clients expressed a lack of control over scheduling and other aspects of service delivery. Case managers may overestimate the flexibility of their care plans, or they may find themselves in a conflict in which they must choose between the needs and values of the agency and those of elderly clients (Hennessy, 1989; Clemens et al., 1994; Kane and Caplan, 1990).

Conclusion

As public policy places increased importance on case management as the coordinating function of the entire long-term care system, case managers find themselves pushed and pulled among competing values and environmental demands in the long-term care decision-making process. Their service as client advocates, traditionally the case managers' central role, may be substantially constricted by the changing environment. Support of client autonomy and protection of client safety, important bases for the philosophy of practice and professional ethics, require reexamination and renewal, tasks that are taken up by Agich (Chap. 6) and Collopy (Chap. 7) later in this volume.

REFERENCES

Abramson, J., and Mizrahi, T. (1987). Strategies for enhancing collaboration between social workers and physicians. *Social Work in Health Care,* 12: 1–21.

Agich, G.J. (1990). Reassessing autonomy in long-term care. *Hastings Center Report,* 20: 12–17.

American Nurses Association. (1976). *The Code for Nurses.* Kansas City, Mo.: American Nurses Association.

American Nurses Association. (1988). *Nursing Case Management.* Kansas City, Mo.: American Nurses Association.

Applebaum, R.A., and Austin, C.D. (1990). *Long-Term Care Case Management: Design and Evaluation.* New York: Springer Publishing Co.

Austin, C.D., Low, L., Roberts, E., and O'Connor, K. (1985). *Case Management:*

A Critical Review. Seattle: University of Washington, Institute on Aging.

Avorn, J., and Langer, E. (1982). Induced disability in nursing home patients: A controlled trial. *Journal of the American Geriatrics Society, 30:* 397–400.

Beauchamp, T.L., and Childress, J.F. (1994). *Principles of Biomedical Ethics,* 4th ed. New York: Oxford University Press.

Biggs, A.J. (1990). Family caregiver versus nursing assessments of elderly self-care abilities. Biggs Elderly Self-Care Assessment Tool. *Journal of Gerontological Nursing, 16(8):* 11–16.

Brody, B. (1993). Case managers and eccentric clients. In R.A. Kane and A.L. Caplan (eds.), *Ethical Conflicts in the Management of Home Care: The Case Manager's Dilemma,* pp. 85–93. New York: Springer Publishing Co.

Callahan, D. (1987). *Setting Limits.* New York: Simon and Schuster.

Camp, L. (1988). A comparison of nurses' recorded assessments of pain with perceptions of pain as described by cancer patients. *Cancer Nursing, 11(4):* 237–243.

Churchill, L. (1988). Should we ration health care by age? *Journal of the American Geriatrics Society, 36:* 644–657.

Clemens E. (in press, 1994). Multiple perceptions of discharge planning in one urban hospital. *Health and Social Work.*

Clemens, E., Wetle, T., Feltes, M., Crabtree, B., and Dubitzky, D. (1994). Contradictions in case management: Client-centered theory and directive practice. *Journal of Aging and Health, 6:* 70–88.

Collopy, B. (1993). The burden of beneficence. In R.A. Kane and A.L. Caplan (eds.), *Ethical Conflicts in the Management of Home Care: The Case Manager's Dilemma,* pp. 93–100. New York: Springer Publishing Co.

Collopy, B.J., Dubler, N.N., and Zuckerman, C. (1990). The ethics of home care: Autonomy and accommodation. *Hastings Center Report, 20*(Special Supplement): 1–16.

Coulton, C., Dunkle, R., Goode, R.A., and MacKintoch, J. (1982). Discharge planning as a decision making process. *Health and Social Work, 7:* 253–261.

Davitz, L.J. (1969). Nurses' inferences of suffering. *Nursing Research, 18:* 100–107.

Dubler, N. (1988). Improving the discharge planning process: Distinguishing between coercion and choice. *Gerontologist, 28*(Special Supplement): 76–81.

Feltes, M., Wetle, T., Clemens, E., Crabtree, B., Dubitzky, D., and Kerr, M. (1994). Case managers and physicians: Communication and perceived problems. *Journal of the American Geriatrics Society, 42:* 5–10.

Fanale, J., Keenan, J., Hepburn, K.W., and von Sternberg, T. (1991). Care management. *Journal of the American Geriatrics Society, 39*: 431–437.

Fox, P. (1981). *Long-Term Care: Background and Future Directions. Publication No. HCFA 81-20047*. Washington, D.C.: U.S. Government Printing Office.

Gadow, S. (1980). Medicine, ethics, and the elderly. *Gerontologist, 20*: 680–685.

Greenfield, S., Blanco, D.M., Elashoff, R.M., and Ganz, P.A. (1987). Patterns of care related to age of breast cancer patients. *Journal of the American Medical Association, 257*: 2766–2770.

Hennessy, C. (1989). Autonomy and risk: The role of client wishes in community-based long-term care. *Gerontologist, 29*: 633–639.

Huntington, J. (1981). *Social Work and General Medical Practice: Collaboration or Conflict*. London: George Allen University.

Iris, M.A. (1988). Guardianship and the elderly: A multiperspective view of the decisionmaking process. *Gerontologist, 28*(Supplement): 39–45.

Kane, R.A. (1988a). Case management in health care settings. In M. Weil, J. Karls, and Associates, (eds.), *Case Management in Human Service Practice*, pp. 170–201. San Francisco: Jossey-Bass.

Kane, R.A. (1988b). Case management: Ethical pitfalls on the road to high-quality managed care. *Quality Review Bulletin, 14*: 161–166.

Kane, R.A., and Caplan, A.L. (eds.). (1990). *Everyday Ethics: Resolving Dilemmas in Nursing Home Life*. New York: Springer Publishing Co.

Kane, R.A., and Caplan, A.L. (eds.). (1993). *Ethical Conflicts in the Management of Home Care: The Case Manager's Dilemma*. New York: Springer Publishing Co.

Kane, R.A., Penrod, J.D., and Kivnick, H.Q. (1993). Ethics and case management: Preliminary results of an empirical study. In R.A. Kane and A.L. Caplan (eds.), *Ethical Conflicts in the Management of Home Care: The Case Manager's Dilemma*, 7–25. New York: Springer Publishing Co.

Kane, R.A., and Thomas, C.A. (1993). What is case management, and why does it raise ethical issues? In R.A. Kane and A.L. Caplan (eds.), *Ethical Conflicts in the Management of Home Care: The Case Manager's Dilemma*, pp. 3–6. New York: Springer Publishing Co.

Kapp, M. (1987). Interprofessional relationships in geriatrics: Ethical and legal considerations. *Gerontologist, 27*: 547–552.

Katz, J. (1984). *The Silent World of Doctor and Patient*. New York: Free Press.

Kautzer, K. (1988). Empowering nursing home residents: A case study of "Living is for the Elderly," an activist nursing home organization. In S. Reinharz and G.D. Rowles (eds.), *Qualitative Gerontology*, pp. 163–183. New York: Springer Publishing Co.

Kerson, T. (1980). *Medical Social Work: The Pre-Professional Paradox*. New York: Irvington.

Langer, E.J. (1983). *The Psychology of Control*. Beverly Hills, Calif.: Sage Publications.

Leutz, W., Greenberg, J., Abrahams, R., Prottas, J., Diamond, L.M., and Gruenberg, L. (1985). *Changing Health Care for an Aging Society*. Lexington, Mass.: Lexington Books.

Levkoff, S., and Wetle, T. (1989). Clinical decision making in care of the elderly. *Journal of Aging and Health, 1*: 83–101.

Lidz, C.W., Appelbaum, P.S., and Meisel, A. (1988). Two models of implementing the idea of informed consent. *Archives of Internal Medicine, 148*: 1385–1389.

Lo, B., McLeod, G., and Saika, G. (1986). Patient attitudes to discussing life-sustaining treatment. *Archives of Internal Medicine, 146*: 1613–1615.

Lo, B., Saika, G., and Strull, W. (1985). Do not resuscitate decisions: A prospective study at three teaching hospitals. *Archives of Internal Medicine, 145*: 1115–1117.

Lynn-McHale, D., and Belinger, A. (1988). Need satisfaction levels of family members of critical care patients and accuracy of nurses' perceptions. *Heart and Lung, 17*: 447–453.

Makadon, H. (1985). Nurses and physicians: Prospects for collaboration. *Annals of Internal Medicine, 103*: 134.

MaloneBeach, E., Zarit, S., and Spore, D. (1992). Caregivers' perceptions of case management and community-based services: Barriers to service use. *Journal of Applied Gerontology, 11*: 146–159.

McCullough, L.B. (1984). Medical care for elderly patients of diminished competence: An ethical analysis. *Journal of the American Geriatrics Society, 32*: 150–153.

Mizrahi, T., and Abramson, J. (1985). Sources of strain between physicians and social workers: Implications for social workers in the health care setting. *Social Work in Health Care, 10*(3): 33–51.

Moxley, D. (1989). *The Practice of Case Management in the Human Services*. Beverly Hills, Calif.: Sage Publications.

Moxley, D.P., and Buzas, L. (1989). Perceptions of case management services for elderly people. *Health and Social Work, 14*: 196–203.

Mullaly, Z. (1988). The application of a social work perspective: A shared social worker-doctor responsibility. *Australian Social Work, 41*: 5.

National Association of Social Workers (1990). NASW Code of Ethics and Professional Standards. Silver Spring, Md.: National Association of Social Workers.

Newquist, D., Hickey, T., and Rakowski, W. (1980). Health assessments of older adults by their families. Paper presented to the annual meeting of the Gerontological Society, San Diego.

Rakowski, W., and Hickey, T. (1979). Family resource persons and geriatric clinic outpatients: Examining the congruence of health beliefs and temporal perspective. Paper presented to the 107th annual meeting of the American Public Health Association, New York, N.Y.

Rodin, J. (1986). Aging and health: Effects of the sense of control. *Science, 233*: 1271–1276.

Schensul, J.J., Torres, M., and Wetle, T. (1992). *Educational Materials and Innovative Dissemination Strategies: Alzheimer's Disease among Puerto Rican Elderly.* Hartford, Conn.: Institute for Community Research.

Simon-Rusinowitz, L., and Hofland, B.F. (1993). Adopting a disability approach to home care services for older adults. *Gerontologist, 33*: 159–167.

Strull, W.M., Lo, B., and Charles, G. (1984). Do patients want to participate in medical decision making? *Journal of the American Medical Association, 252*: 2990–2994.

Tauer, C.A. (1993). Risks and choices: When is paternalism justified? In R.A. Kane and A. Caplan (eds.), *Ethical Conflicts in Management of Health Care: The Case Manager's Dilemma,* pp. 45–55. New York: Springer Publishing Co.

Weil, M., Karis, J., and Associates. (1985). *Case Management in Human Service Practices.* San Francisco: Jossey-Bass.

Wetle, T. (1987). Age as a risk factor for inadequate treatment. *Journal of the American Medical Association, 258*: 516.

Wetle, T. (1988). Ethical issues. In J.W. Rowe and R.W. Besdine (eds.), *Geriatric Medicine,* pp. 75–88. Boston: Little, Brown and Co.

Wetle, T. (1991). Resident decision making and quality of life in the frail elderly. In J.E. Birren, J.E. Lubben, J.C. Rowe, and D.E. Deutchman (eds.), *The Concept and Measurement of Quality of Life in the Frail Elderly,* pp. 315–334. New York: Academic Press.

Wetle, T., Crabtree, B., Clemens, E., Dubitzky, D., Eslami, M., and Kerr, M. (1991). Balancing safety and autonomy: Defining and living with acceptable risk. *Gerontologist, 31*(2): 237.

Wetle, T., Cwikel, J., and Levkoff, S. (1988). Geriatric medical decisions: Factors influencing allocation of scarce resources and the decision to withhold treatment. *Gerontologist, 28*: 336.

Wetle, T., Dubitzky, D., Feltes, M., Clemens, E., Crabtree, B., and Winsemius, D. (1992). Case managers and elderly clients: Concordance in perceptions of control, information sharing and self esteem. *Gerontologist, 32*: 46–47.

Wetle, T., Levkoff, S., Cwikel, J., and Rosen, A. (1988). Nursing home resident participation in medical decisions: Perceptions and preferences. *Gerontologist, 28*: 32–38.

Williams, O.J. (1993). When is being equal unfair? In R.A. Kane and A.L. Caplan (eds.), *Ethical Conflicts in the Management of Home Care: The Case Manager's Dilemma*, pp. 206–215. New York: Springer Publishing Co.

CHAPTER FIVE

Decision Making, Care Plans, and Life Plans
in Long-Term Care: Can Case Managers Take Account
of Clients' Values and Preferences?

Rosalie A. Kane

Professionals necessarily intrude into the decision making of older people contemplating or receiving long-term care (LTC) in the range of settings described by Nancy Wilson (Chap. 3) in this volume. Nurses, social workers, and physicians advise, recommend, counsel, and persuade persons seeking assistance to adopt various plans. In the all-too-telling language that has become commonplace in U.S. hospitals, they "place" older people in nursing homes. Often the advice given to older people, especially those in hospitals, is based on a brief acquaintance only, and often the hospital discharge planner is as preoccupied with timely release of a hospital bed as with the best interests of the individual (Abramson, 1988).

As indicated in previous chapters (Wilson, Chap. 3; Wetle, Chap. 4), a relatively new long-term care professional, called case manager or care coordinator, has emerged in the last decade or so with responsibilities to assist individuals and families in making care plans (Applebaum and Austin, 1990; Quinn, 1993). Typically drawn from the ranks of social workers or nurses, case managers are expected to act as advocates for elderly and disabled clients. Ideally, they are free from the conflicts of interest of the hospital discharge planner. Often they are completely separated from direct service delivery so that they can package a service plan without considering their own self-interest as potential providers. When case managers have authority to purchase services using public funds, they base their recommendations on elaborate and standardized assessments of the older person's physical status and social situation. The ultimate choices are meant to be left to clients (assuming the clients are adjudged competent), but case managers' suggestions take into account the adequacy of care and the likely safety of the client under the best scenario they can envisage for care at home. That is, before recommending care at home rather than in a nursing home, they consider, often with considerable anguish, the availability of assistance in the geographic area, the program rules governing the amount of care that can be directly purchased, the availability of private client resources to purchase services, and the amount and type of volunteered help from families and friends (Kane and Caplan, 1993). Then, for clients living outside nursing homes, case managers authorize, allocate, and monitor particular services, sometimes making minute adjustments in the amount, timing, and nature of the help the client receives.

Thus, long-term care professionals, and particularly case managers, regularly make judgments and decisions that affect the lives of older people with functional impairments and their families sometimes in intimate and sometimes in dramatic ways. This chapter explores whether it is feasible and desirable for such professionals to make systematic efforts to learn the values of their clients and incorporate such information into the care plans they make. Would such a refocusing lead to improved care plans or to improved decisions? Can professionals, armed with knowledge of client values and preferences, assist their clients in making better decisions? If values and preferences are brought to the services and discussed among clients, family members, and professionals, might this redress the balance of power among the long-term care decision-making participants?

Background
The Elusive Nature of Long-Term Care Decisions

As Laurence McCullough and Nancy Wilson state in their introductory chapter, long-term care decision making involves multiple parties with specific interests and obligations. As they and their colleagues point out in Chapter 11 of this volume, long-term care decisions can rarely be encapsulated into clear-cut decision moments as has been done, perhaps artificially, for acute-care decisions about particular surgical or medical treatments. The model of the rational decision makers who gather all relevant information and use it to reach decisions that maximize their well-being is an economist's or a philosopher's fantasy.

Putting research wisdom into practice regarding long-term care decision making is, therefore, almost doomed by the paucity of trustworthy data. Below is a list of difficulties.

1. Decisions are made in a social context. In long-term care, both the older person who perceives a need for help and family members who may decide to provide care have decisions to make. One decides whether to accept care, the other whether to give it. Each is influenced by the other, sometimes by explicit advice and sometimes by inferences about what is important to the other. We have little research about this interaction.

2. Decisions are dynamic, although present decisions are constrained by previous decisions. Even the decision about nursing home admission, which is never routine from the perspective of the person who is to become a resident, is not irrevocable.

3. Decisions may not lead to action or change. When a conscious decision is made not to relocate to receive long-term care or not to accept outside help, an observer cannot readily see that decision or examine its results. But research (Brody, Kleban, and Leibowitz, 1984) identified a phenomenon of immobilization, when older people simply failed to engage in considering whether they should or should not move into specialized housing. In operational terms, however, it is difficult to distinguish between a decision not to take action and avoidance of any decision making at all; in both situations, no change occurs.

4. Little is known about the natural course of decision making (e.g., when people perceive that they begin trying to decide something, when decision making has ended, or, for that matter, whether any conscious decision making takes place).

5. Decisions are blurry. In long-term care, for example, interrelated decisions may be needed or made regarding personal care, housing, finances, family responsibilities, and advance directives. Isolating the topic of decisions for research purposes is difficult.

6. From a researcher's perspective, studies of decision making are rendered difficult by lack of agreed-upon terminology to define and classify decisions themselves, i.e., the independent variable. Presumably, decisions vary not only by topical content, but by their importance, the degree of conscious attention they are given, elapsed time in making the decision, the number of alternatives considered, the kind and amount of information sought and received, and the influence of other people.

7. Authorities disagree about what makes a decision good. Objective criteria could be developed that concentrate either on outcomes judged a priori to be good, outcomes judged good by the client, or on the process of the decision. Thus, studies of decision making flounder on definitions

of the dependent variables—the measures of outcomes of decision making. In their classic study of decision making under psychological stress, Irving Janis and Leon Mann (1977) suggest that a good decision is one that is made after a rational appraisal of available alternatives, hampered by neither discouraged attitudes nor time pressures, and that a good decision minimizes "post-decisional regret." Even if people are unhappy with their lives after the decision, the theory goes, they will be sanguine that they made the best choice at the time.

8. Once people make decisions, they try to live with those decisions. After buying a home or a car, for example, the decision makers tend to justify their choices after the fact and become impervious to other homes or cars still on the market. Thus, as Janis and Mann (1977) also point out, real satisfaction with decisions reached is hard to distinguish from the human tendency to "bolster the least undesirable alternative."

Given the murkiness surrounding the study of long-term care decisions, proving that explicit surfacing of clients' values and preferences changes such decisions would clearly be difficult. However, the fact remains that case managers purport to apply their knowledge and understanding of clients to assisting them in what is often difficult decision making. Perhaps because of the very complexity and elusiveness of long-term care decisions, conscious attention to values and preferences among those who have decisions to make and those who try to help would be beneficial to the older person receiving help.

Problems in Long-Term Care Decision Making

Long-term care decisions may be hard to isolate or to evaluate with research tools. Yet, we do know that the context under which older people make long-term care decisions often is pressured and inimical to informed choice (Agich, Chap. 6). Older people with functional impairments may need to make many difficult and interrelated decisions at the same time that they recognize a need for long-term care. These may be about medical care procedures; about home renovation; about relocation to a group living environment; about future relationships and roles in their family, including accepting care from family members; about whether to purchase or accept paid help at home; about money matters (e.g., sale of property, divestment of assets to become eligible for subsidized care programs); and about a permanent or temporary stay in a nursing home. Such important decisions about their care and their lives are typically made without adequate information or reflection. Older persons may, in fact, be too physically ill or debilitated to actively engage in decision making. They may not know how or have time to search for information. Consider the following:

1. Long-term care decisions are often made in a hurry and under stress. This is particularly true if the older person is in a hospital or if the perceived need for a decision has been precipitated by a health crisis that has caused the family to gather around.

2. Long-term care decisions are often made without consulting the person most involved, let alone providing him or her with information needed to reach a decision.

3. Professionals who assist with long-term care decisions often have extraneous incentives and pressures. The hospital discharge planner may need to free up the hospital bed. The case manager for community care may have established good relationships with particular vendors or may have a commitment to send some business their way.

4. Some, but by no means all, older people have diminished capacity to make decisions. However, the pervasive image in many health care settings is that all or most older people are cognitively impaired. Professionals sometimes consult family members before or instead of consulting the older person.

5. Long-term care clients and their families often describe actions that are taken without conscious decision making (Thuras et al., 1992). This may be the result of doing what comes naturally (of course I would take care of my husband), or of drift (my daughter lived nearby and before I knew it, she was coming every day). In some situations, decisions may be actively avoided, when, for instance, there is more interest in maintaining the stability of relationships than in making deliberate decisions.

6. Ellen Langer (1989) describes decisions that are made on a type of "automatic pilot," rather than what she calls "mindfully." Mindlessness or lack of conscious decision making may occur because of limited categories or mind sets and automatic behavior that dulls consciousness. Familiar contexts and perceptions of strained resources can dull professionals into mindlessness. Unfortunately, case managers, hospital discharge planners, and others who advise elderly people about long-term care options are prone to this phenomenon, making them less than adequate decision counselors.

Later in this volume George Agich (Chap. 6) makes a distinction between nodal and interstitial decisions. The former are the type of clear-cut decisions about a course of action that are readily analyzed by ethicists, whereas the latter are the repetitive, daily decisions that are intertwined with ordinary life. While it would be tempting to suggest that the nodal decisions are unlikely to be on automatic pilot or be made without conscious recognition of the decision maker, no data support that contention. Our own research suggests that it is rare for a portentous decision, such as entering a nursing home, to be made without conscious deliberation by those most concerned (Thuras et al., 1992).

Research Findings

Theory and research about human decision making are almost embarrassingly plentiful, yet such a body of knowledge is difficult to fashion into a coherent whole. At least three streams of work are relevant to long-term care decisions of older people and their families.

Learned Helplessness

By now a reliable body of research attests that failure to make decisions or to perceive oneself in control of decisions is dangerous for one's health (Seligman, 1975). Those who perceive that they have no control over decisions affecting their lives are at risk of depression, morbidity, and even mortality. This theory has been tested most in the low-control nursing home environment where during the 1970s researchers demonstrated that adding opportunities for choice and control led to surprisingly impressive benefits (Langer and Rodin, 1976; Mercer and Kane, 1979; Schulz, 1976).

Psychological Stress

Janis and his colleagues (Janis and Mann, 1977) repeatedly demonstrated that people making decisions under stress often fail to examine all reasonable alternatives, taking into account for each course of action the practical consequences for themselves and those they care about and the likely consequences for how the decision makers expect they will feel about themselves and others will feel about them. This kind of decision making, dubbed "vigilant," is short-circuited if the decision maker lacks hope that a good decision can be reached or believes that urgent time pressures exist. The preconditions for the good decision, which Janis defines as one where postdecisional regret is minimized, are often absent for the long-term care client.

Bounded Rationality and Framing

Not being computers, human minds are capable of examining only a relatively small number of variables simultaneously. The human mind is also suggestible. Different conclusions may be reached for precisely the same problem based on the way questions are framed and how vivid various alternatives are in the mind of the decider (Tversky and Kahneman, 1981; Tversky, Sattath, and Slovic, 1988). This places the onus on professionals who help frame problems and alternative solutions for the elderly decision maker. These phenomena have so far largely been studied in laboratory situations with hypothetical problems. In the real world, we assume that decision makers presumably reframe problems and are influenced in this process. For example, how professionals present information influences what people remember (Tymchuk et al., 1988).

To illustrate in the area of long-term care, professionals may emphasize the risks of remaining at home alone, while ignoring any risks associated with entering a nursing home. Similarly, they may highlight a negative outcome, such as falling, versus a positive one, such as independence. They may underscore a client's need for "twenty-four-hour care" as a reason to consider a nursing home, leaving the client with the impression that the average nursing home provides twenty-four-hour care. In fact, the actual amount of care from nursing personnel for nursing home residents averages seventy minutes a day, and the average amount of time from licensed nursing personnel, such as RNs and LPNs, averages less than ten minutes a day. It might be possible to replicate that amount of care for the same price at home, though without the potential to meet unscheduled needs. Experiments on the effects of how problems are framed are usually done with hypothetical scenarios (to hold constant the stimulus); little work is available to describe how the alternative choices are framed in real-life settings and with what results.

Assessment and Care Planning

Long-term care professionals do more than assist their clients with dramatic decisions. They also help arrange the myriad details of everyday life for long-term care clients. As stated above, case managers often can authorize or purchase services for the client. Thus, they make numerous small decisions (one hopes, in conjunction with the older person) to determine what kind of care to arrange, when, and from whom. The tools for this professional decision making are the comprehensive, multidimensional, functional assessment and the care plan flowing from it.

Assessment

Though varying from each other in detail, comprehensive long-term care assessments have evolved into recognizable procedures. They take substantial time and characteristically touch similar bases. Through such assessments, professionals attempt to reliably characterize an older person's physical health, functional abilities, cognitive abilities, psychological states, social well-being, and past and current use of formal services and family help. For community-dwelling elders, the assessment sometimes also examines the extent to which family members are available for or stressed by caregiving roles. The battery of questions may lead to scores by which professionals compare older people on these parameters and to notation of issues relevant for care planning. The comprehensive assessment may then be used to determine eligibility or need for services, to tailor service plans to meet individual needs, to establish priorities for scarce services, and to allocate services.

A minimum data set (MDS) has been mandated to be collected for all nursing home residents, and these data, in turn, are expected to inform care plans for nursing home residents (Morris et al., 1990). In most states, case managers use one or more similar comprehensive assessment tools to assess potential home care clients, to allocate services to them, to monitor the client's ongoing progress, and to readjust service levels and types.

With few exceptions, these comprehensive assessments pay little attention to the values or preferences of the person assessed. The nursing home MDS does have a section on customary routines in the year prior to admission, which is completed on the first admission only. On a yes or no basis, it records customary routines, such as staying up after 9 P.M., leaving home at least once a week, staying busy with hobbies, preferring particular foods, eating between meals, using alcoholic beverages, preferring a shower over bathing, attending church regularly, daily contact with relatives, friends, or animals, and involvement in group activities. This portion of the assessment is not particularly reliable; it is also not informative about the specifics of what is important to the new resident.

Nor is there any clarity about how the information should be used to individualize nursing home care. Most state assessment batteries for community care completely ignore the subject of client values or limit their attention to questions about whether the client has made advance directives of various kinds.

Care Planning

The lack of attention to client values would be less disturbing were care plans less obtrusive, all-encompassing, and defining in the lives of long-term care clients. After all, accountants, attorneys, physicians, and architects often make technical recommendations and provide technical services without much understanding of their clients as persons. Clients are expected to weigh such advice against their understanding of their own values. Generally, the professionals and clients have a common frame of reference to understand the encounter, and generally the power of the professional is circumscribed.

In contrast, a nursing home care plan becomes a guideline for the life of the nursing home resident. It describes not only medications and nursing procedures, but details of when and how the resident will be dressed, bathed, and helped in and out of bed. It includes what the resident is allowed to eat, whether alcoholic beverages are permitted, and whether the resident can be unsupervised. Moreover, observations are regularly made about residents on whether they finish the food on their plates, their weight, their moods, their visitors, their toileting schedule, which serve to objectify residents and narrow them to the sum of these observed items. Such data feed back into care plans, and life by care plan is a sterile affair. Janet Tulloch (in press, 1995), a nursing home resident, activist, and writer, refers to the care plan as "an instrument of terror" because of its powerful role in a resident's daily life.

A care plan for a home care client typically outlines the kinds of tasks that will be performed in the client's home, divides responsibility between family members and paid caregivers, and sometimes itemizes the concrete tasks in-home workers will perform (e.g., prepare a meal, do the laundry, walk the dog, help the client to the toilet). For example, the care plan may indicate that a personal care worker will come to the home three days a week to perform certain tasks and that the client will go to a day care center two days a week. Sometimes the details of timing and tasks will be planned by the case manager and sometimes a home care provider will flesh out the detail within the general prescriptions and cost caps the case managers establish. In contrast to a nursing home care plan, the case manager's care plan is less likely to dictate the client's entire life, because home care providers do not exert the same degree of control. However, if the client is really disabled, the home care plan may establish the parameters of his or her life, dictating the timing of routines and establishing the presence of a helper in the client's home.

Once a care plan is established the case manager monitors the situation, responding to requests for changes from both client and care providers and reassessing the client to determine whether the plan is adequate to meet the client's needs. Typically, case managers recommend a nursing home if they deem that care cannot be provided safely or adequately in the home setting within the available financial resources (which must be less than the cost of a nursing home for a comparable client).

What Goes Wrong

Several observations made by and of case management programs suggest the need for values assessment.

Cookie cutter care plans. Despite the specificity and comprehensiveness of the typical assessment, care plans tend to show little variation or creativity. This can be true even when programs permit the case managers to purchase just about anything or any service for their clients (Frankfather, Smith, and Caro, 1981). One wonders if plans would be more responsive if case managers knew their clients better.

Client refusal of service. Although the scarcity of community-based services and of funds to purchase these services is well known, commentators often do not recognize the propensity of clients to refuse those services that are offered and to accept less than the professional believes is necessary. Why are services so often a "hard sell"? One speculation is that they are offered in undesired forms or that the clients perceive that they have too little control over the original plan and the ongoing changes.

Safety above all. Rhetoric holds that case managers should revere the autonomy of the clients they serve and act as their advocates. However, in practice, concerns about a client's safety tend to override other values (Kane, Penrod, and Kivnick, 1994; Wetle, Chap. 4). One wonders if this situation could be alleviated if case managers better understood their clients' values, if family members better understood their relatives' values, and if clients could better articulate their own values. Later in this volume, Bart Collopy (Chap. 7) offers another strategy, namely, seeing safety and independence as two ends of a single continuum.

Toward Formal Values "Assessment"
Why Inquire about Clients' Values?

The discussion above argues that those who assess the functional well being of older people and plan their care cannot be counted upon to be aware of the values and preferences of their clients. Moral arguments for gathering this information are usually framed around respect for personal autonomy. If case managers and other long-term care professionals know more about their clients' values, they can take them into account in making care plans. Arthur Caplan (1992), Joan Gibson (1990), and David Doukas and McCullough (1991) have argued that such knowledge could be useful to guide professionals in working with clients who become cognitively impaired; thus, Caplan urges doing a "values baseline" and Gibson, as well as Doukas and McCullough, a "values history" to make individual values explicit while it is still possible.

Arguably, however, knowledge of clients' values and preferences is equally, if not more, important in providing the basis for respect for the autonomy of persons who are cognitively intact. Gibson argues convincingly that people cannot readily articulate their own values in a way that informs their personal decision making unless they have participated in an effort to explore them systematically. This argument suggests that encouraging clients to discover and order their preferences enhances client autonomy in the sense of positive freedom; it provides a forum for bringing their own values into the forefront and emphasizes that they do have choices. The process of exploring values is, thus, considered just as important as the list ultimately produced.

Agich (Chap. 6) suggests in this volume and elsewhere (1993) that autonomy in long-term care conveys more than just self-direction. It also involves consistency, so that the sense of self of the person receiving care remains intact. Since much long-term care, especially in institutional settings, seems to attack and erode the very sense of identity of clients (Tobin, 1991) and their autonomy (Lidz, Fischer, and Arnold, 1992), attention to individual values and preferences would seem a corrective in the direction of increased respect for autonomy.

Most importantly, attention to clients' values, if accompanied by a proper spirit of inquiry and modesty, might provide a corrective to expanding pressures to apply "science" to human service disciplines. It is that impulse that makes some planners believe that the "correct" plan can be ordered for each long-term care client's life if only the right information is collected and analyzed. Robert Bellah (1982) offers a contrasting view in his contention that: "The purpose of practice is not to produce or control anything but to discover through mutual discussion and reflection between free citizens the most appropriate ways, under present conditions, of living the ethically good life" (p. 36).

Why Be Cautious about Values Assessment?

Several arguments can be advanced *against* routine inquiry about the values and preferences of clients. To my mind, none of these are arguments against proceeding, but they do suggest safeguards to be built into the process.

Hubris. Comprehensive assessments already "commodify" clients to some extent, reducing them to the sum of the items observed in the assessment. Some might argue that attempting to encapsulate the values of the client is the crowning audacity, doomed to failure and likely to lead to a complacent, but erroneous belief that professionals can know everything about a client. Taken to an extreme, this concern might suggest that values should remain a zone of privacy for the clients. More reasonably, however, application of this caution would direct that case managers inquire about clients' values repeatedly and that they review their understandings with clients in a continuous way as care plans are revised over time. It also argues for a separate protocol on values and preferences that is not contained within the all-inclusive comprehensive assessment.

False promises. Another concern is that those who assess values and preferences are implicitly promising to honor them. This argument is made by those who believe that few choices are possible, given resource constraints and inflexible systems of care. This concern seems somewhat disingenuous. If, indeed, the services we offer to elderly people with disabilities are inimical to their preferences and change their lives in ways that they perceive as negative, we are obliged to improve those services. It makes the situation no worse if case managers listen to their clients tell them about what they value. What is added, as in the explicit sharing of secrets, is the added discomfort for case managers whose clients now "know that they know" how bad it is. With explicit attention, a creative case manager has some chance of tailoring plans to better fit the client even in relatively inflexible service systems. Furthermore, aggregate information can be gathered about the extent to which client preferences are met across a group of clients. This permits case managers to move from "case to cause" using clients' views in efforts to change policies and increase options.

Indeed, making creative, responsive care plans takes practice and builds on interest in and understanding of the client's values. There may be more room for individual attention than case managers recognize. Care planning occurs within care planning, resembling the nested dolls that serve as children's toys. After an initial decision about nursing home care versus community care come decisions about the broad types of community care to choose and choices of particular agencies to provide it. After that and perhaps more important to the client are choices about the timing and specific tasks done by care workers. Also relevant is how well the style of the personal care worker coincides with the client's preferences, reflected in the choice of an individual worker or helper. Finally, the care plan could encompass plans and goals that pertain to the case manager's own activities and style while working with the client.

Misuse of the assessment. Some critics suggest that if values are assessed, professionals may use this information in a rote way, consulting the record instead of consulting the client as plans are modified over time. Some worry that case managers will get the answers wrong and then act on those wrong answers. However, this seems overscrupulous because presently many case managers act on no answers at all. If they do not ask about values, they are likely to guess. The best informant is the client. Discussions about values with the client, if done with sufficient time and serious interest in the answers, are likely to sensitize both clients and case managers to the importance of these issues and the desirability of revisiting them.

Content and Format of Assessment

Vast amounts of information could be collected on client values and preferences, but this would fast become impracticable. Some of the areas that seem relevant to long-term care include the following: personal privacy and living environment; daily routines; preferred social activities; family roles in care; life plans and projects; pain and discomfort; personal safety and protection; death and dying; religion and spirituality; and use of financial resources. This laundry list manifestly ranges from the mundane to the sublime, and many pieces of discreet information could be placed under each heading. In the course of this exploration, case managers will also learn the extent to which this particular client puts a high value on control and planning itself.

Determining whether any topic has importance for the client is only part of the task. It would then be necessary to explore the details. What is it about, for example, privacy or religious involvement, that is important to that client? For example, our own pilot work shows that clients who rated privacy as very important had different elaborations on what it meant to them: one wanted to spend periods of time alone; one wanted to protect bodily privacy; one was concerned about privacy in financial transactions; and one did not like other people to be able to look through her possessions. Had we just asked the respondents to rate the importance of privacy to them, we would have been deprived of the client's particular meaning. Similarly, there were those for whom the ordering of daily routines was unimportant (who described themselves as flexible), but for those who did place importance on their rituals of daily life, there were many variations in content. One man explained that he liked to get up, shave, read the paper, and take a shower, in that order. Others stress the importance of particular kinds of food. Such detail is relevant to the timing of personal care assistance and the tasks the assistant is asked to do. A guided discussion of this nature, of course, reveals what is salient to the client in ways that go beyond the direct question. For example, one woman mentioned her dog in every other answer. Feeding the dog and letting him out in the yard were important parts of her daily routine, and the dog was integral to her plans. It would be impractical to ask about every conceivable matter of importance to clients in relation to their activities and their environment, but it is feasible to use a few broad triggering questions to identify these themes.

Thus, we do not advocate that case managers or nursing home personnel use rating scales or ranking strategies to assess their clients' values. Similarly, we do not advocate taking measures of particular values off the shelf, however excellent their provenance. Measures are available in abundance to gauge the presence of particular values, such as conservatism or religiosity. First, such a strategy is impractical because of the time involved and the huge number of values that can be tapped. Second, the questions will be alien and without face validity to the clients unless linked to their care. Third, after we learn that the client is a 15 on an 18-point conservatism scale, we still would not know the meaning of that information for the client's care plan. And, finally, the purpose of this approach is to begin a process in which clients think about their values in relationship to their care, the case manager thinks about them as well, and they begin to talk together. These are the basis of the preventive ethics strategy described in Chapter 11 of this volume.

Mechanics of Attending to Values

Over the last few years, we have held preliminary discussions with case managers about whether and how client values could be appraised and incorporated into their work. We have also piloted various ways to ask about client values. Although many case managers like the idea, enthusiasm is tempered by a range of practical reservations. In addition to the objections already cited, other logistical issues are raised.

Time and timing. Not all case managers are universally enthusiastic about this approach. Even those who felt they had gained new insight into their clients through this process raised questions about the amount of time such assessments would take. Some suggested that the values assessment be postponed until the reassessment six months later "when there is not so much care planning to do." Some were confident that they could learn all this content in the course of the regular assessment with just a bit more attention to probing. For example, they could learn about feelings and preferences regarding care from family members and from strangers during the part of the assessment that dealt with the amount and source of current assistance received, and they could learn about the values of the client around daily routines at the time that ability to perform ADL is examined.

Arguably, one should begin this process before the client's first care plan is developed (rather than have verdict first, trial afterward). It is also important to return to the assessment and its content at subsequent meetings. And diffusing the content throughout the entire comprehensive assessment makes the values assessment lose its integrity as a product as well as a process. Case managers, clients, and families should be able to return to the value-based material and work with it.

Who should explore values? In some large case management pro-grams, initial assessments are done by designated staff who only perform comprehensive assessments. Another person, assigned to be case manager, takes that assessment and without repeating it (though some "spot-checks" are said to be done) meets with the client to develop the care plan. It would seem best that the case manager who will have the ongoing relationship begin the values conversations, since the very act of asking and hearing the responses is meant to have an effect on the case manager's thinking. By the same token, it would not be advisable to hire a psychologist to perform all values assessments for all clients. This kind of distancing would defeat the spirit of values assessment.

Where should values information be kept? As envisaged here, the values assessment is a working document to help case managers gain understanding and to help clients gain self-understanding. The information so gained does not lend itself to being computerized and added to a client's care profile. Yet, surely the information should be written down and retained. Certainly, it could also be the basis for discussions among case managers at care planning conferences. One possibility is that the client also be given a copy of the case manager's summary notes. It goes without saying that the case manager should inform the client about any contemplated use of the values assessment (and the entire assessment). Some case managers believe that values questions are too personal and confidential to be asked and recorded. Yet the routine assessment has questions about incontinence, finances, and depression and other mood states. Something else may be operative in the reluctance to approach values, i.e., case managers may not want that amount of intimacy with their clients.

Family members' values. Case managers point out to us that the values of family members who provide help to their relatives also have weight. Arguably, then, case managers should try systematically to learn something about the relevant values of the relevant family actors. If the family member is also the surrogate decision maker for a client with dementia, his or her values as they relate to the relative's care are the most salient of all. Relevant themes may include the family member's view of family duties and responsibilities perhaps along the lines explored by Jecker (Chap. 8) and Brakman (Chap. 9) in this volume; the family member's own life goals and interests, as described by Arras (Chap. 10);

and various preferences for how the family member's own daily routines and activities are conducted. The case manager could also ask the surrogate about the values of the client, although it is by no means clear what weight the latter should carry in the case of discrepancies.

Demonstration Project
Intervention

In 1993, the University of Minnesota launched a demonstration project, funded by the Retirement Research Foundation, in which case managers in a large program agreed to ask all their clients about their values and preferences. The project is viewed as action research because the investigators are collaborating with personnel at the demonstration site to develop the protocols for the innovation and procedures to use the information in ways that enhance clients' autonomy.

We began with a simple one-page assessment tool in which we asked clients to rate the importance of choice and control for seven issues related to their care. Topics included were: daily routines; social activities, including religious participation; family members whom they wish to be involved or not to be involved in their care; pain and discomfort; future events or projects; privacy; and taking risks versus safety and protection. Once the importance of the topic was rated (as "very important," "somewhat important," or "not important"), the case manager asked for elaboration on what the client saw as important and why. The questions concluded with two open-ended queries: If you could not make decisions about your care, whom would you want to make them and why? What is it that makes you feel most like yourself? These questions were asked upon the initial assessment and any reassessments. When clients were too cognitively impaired to be interviewed, family members were asked about what they thought was important to the client.

Now that about three hundred such interviews have been completed, we have learned several things. First, clients are willing and interested in responding to these questions, though they vary in the amount of detail that they provide. Second, a range of responses can be found. Clients vary from each other in what they consider important areas of choice and control. We also found that clients were able to differentiate their own answers, distinguishing between matters that were more or less important. We certainly found validation for an approach that sought clarification and elaboration on ratings; this was the route to the specific matters that the particular client found paramount. Case man-

agers who piloted the questions with clients they already knew sometimes were surprised by the answers. For instance, one case manager had
expected the client to emphasize the importance of one niece in her life,
but instead the client concentrated on a different relative. One case manager was startled to find that she, the case manager, was the person
whom the client would wish to act as proxy decision maker.

Although we worried that the question "What makes you feel most
like yourself?" might seem a bit metaphysical and abstract to clients, we
found that they seemed to like the question and had ready answers.
Clients sometimes referred to an activity they could no longer pursue,
such as hunting, fishing, or world travel. Most often, however, they
referred to everyday matters. Sample answers included: when I am chat-
ting on the phone; when I go to dinner with my family; when I am
watching the weather channel; and when I am outside on my porch.
Though not a direct question about relative values, our hope was that
this item would provide a glimpse of the client as an authentic person.

Other routines are needed to support the initial assessment. In the
site where the study has been implemented, a large-print brochure is left
with the clients so that they can think about the values issues at leisure.
Case staffing has also been done with a focus on what difference the
client's particular values should make to the care plan. Variations that
may be introduced in this or other settings include a protocol for assessing family values, mechanisms for allowing clients to take informed
risks, and mechanisms for working with provider agencies and individual helpers to foster the care the clients want. The hope is that systematic
attention to values, however mechanistic, will spin off into individualized responses.

Expected Effects

Our plan is to evaluate whether this systematic attention to clients'
values and preferences can really make differences compared to similar
settings in which no special attention is given to them. Given the inertia
and lack of flexibility in systems of care, we were aware of the difficulties
in finding effects. With trepidation, we are hypothesizing the following:

1. Compared to a control group, clients in the values-sensitive environment will be better satisfied with care-planning processes and outcomes.

2. Compared to a control group, family members and case managers

for clients in the values-sensitive environment will be more accurate about the client's values.

3. Compared to a control group, family members and case managers for clients in the values-sensitive environment will be more willing for the client to take risks in order to maximize other preferences.

4. Compared to a control group, care plans of case managers working in the values-sensitive environment will show more variability, flexibility, and creativity.

Bottom Line: Should Caregivers Attend to Clients' Values?

This chapter opened with a discussion of the problems of decision making, emphasizing that decisions are rarely solo or clean-cut; that they are made in social contexts, influenced by many people and by previous decisions; and that subtle differences in the way issues are framed and problems cast will influence the decisions taken. Given this, one could argue that case managers, discharge planners, and other long-term care professionals already have too much power over large and small decisions of their clients and that entrance into the world of the client's values only gives them more.

This issue is related to the discussions that occur around more classic medical decision making about who should apply the patient's utility weights (Kane and Kane, 1982). Some argue that the physician, who will have the information about risks and benefits of various procedures, should find out about the patient's utilities (say, for comfort or a long life) and make a recommendation accordingly. Others suggest that the physician should disclose the risks and benefits to the patient and that the patient should apply personal utilities to the problem. In practice, one suspects that both processes are necessary. The patient may want a formal recommendation from the physician with all the authority it connotes, and the patient may have difficulty applying information about risks and benefits by themselves. But it would be dangerous for a physician to apply utilities outside a dialogue with the patient to be sure that these utilities are clearly understood.

Building on this analogy, in theory, it would be possible to take the position that case managers and other professionals have little business making a wide range of decisions that affect the personal lives of their older clients. One could argue that the professional should simply disclose a wide variety of options at multiple levels (e.g., care at home versus moving to an assisted living setting; care from a talkative, friendly helper versus care from a more taciturn but efficient helper), and the client should select the plan without disclosing his or her own values. Some might even argue that this would be an antidote to the power that has been amassed by professionals. A new Marie Antoinette might say "Let them apply their own utility weights."

On closer inspection, however, the above formulation should be rejected. First, case managers and other long-term care professionals can and do make many judgments and decisions. They do so because of the logistics of their role and the physical condition of the client. Many of the details that could be relevant to the client's values become known only as the care plan unfolds—as it is determined what agencies are available to provide help and what particular workers will be involved in the elder's care. If the professional has entered into a partnership with the client based on the latter's values, surely the balance of power shifts toward greater autonomy of the client. Of course, this strategy is consistent with provision of fuller information to the client and family about the range of options, as well as open-mindedness to entertain a wider range of options.

At some level, the issue of values assessment raises a question of what kind of relationship is envisaged between clients and long-term care professionals, particularly case managers. If the ideal relationship is seen as only formal and impersonal, then clients might be wary of sharing their values. Focus groups of older people receiving home care show that among the qualities clients seek in their workers is that they "care about me as a person, that they care what happens to me." This sense of caring obviously carries a meaning different from providing physical care. (For a discussion of the ethics of personal relationships, see Hardwig, 1989.)

Nancy Eustis has done qualitative studies that suggest that, for the sake of both the hands-on helper and the client, some middle-ground between intimacy and impersonality is needed in the relationship; too personal a relationship destroys boundaries and eventually engenders mutual resentment; too distant a relationship cannot sustain the intimacy of the long-term care encounters (Eustis and Fischer, 1993). Perhaps some similar middle-ground needs to be sought for the relationships between elderly disabled people and their care coordinators in the community or those who care for them in nursing homes. Routine attention to clients' values and preferences may help establish that relationship.

In some senses, the approach advocated here fights fire with fire. I am recommending a routine approach to the personal; a standardized way of coming to know the highly nonstandard wishes and aspirations of elderly clients; a formula to get beyond formula into clients' life stories. If the systematic attention to values and preferences becomes another gimmick, leading to pat answers and formulaic plans, it will be a failure. If it expands personal autonomy for persons with functional impairments that render them dependent and if it allows those who are our clients to maintain a keen sense of self, it will be a success.

REFERENCES

Abramson, J. (1988). Participation of elderly patients in discharge planning. Is self-determination a reality? *Social Work, 33:* 443–448.

Agich, G.J. (1993). *Autonomy and Long-Term Care.* New York: Oxford University Press.

Applebaum, R., and Austin, C. (1990). *Long-term Care Case Management: Design and Evaluation.* New York: Springer Publishing Co.

Banziger, G., and Roush, S. (1983). Nursing home for the birds: A control relevant intervention with bird feeders. *Gerontologist, 23:* 527–531.

Bellah, R.N. (1982). Social science as practical reason. *The Hastings Center Report, 12:* 32–39.

Brody, E.M., Kleban, M.H., and Leibowitz, B. (1984). Intermediate housing for elderly: Satisfaction of those who moved in and those who did not. *Gerontologist, 15:* 350–356.

Caplan, A.L. (1992). Can autonomy be saved. In A.C. Caplan (ed.), *If I Were a Rich Man Could I Buy a Pancreas? and Other Essays on the Ethics of Health Care,* pp. 256–281. Bloomington, Ind.: Indiana University Press.

Doukas, D.J., and McCullough, L.B. (1991). The values history: The evaluation of the patient's values and advance directives. *Journal of Family Practice, 32:* 145–153.

Eustis, N.N., and Fischer, L.R. (1993). Relationships between home care clients and their workers. Implications for quality care. *Gerontologist, 31:* 447–456.

Frankfather, D.L., Smith, M.H., and Caro, F.G. (1981). *Family Care of the Elderly: Public Initiatives and Private Obligations.* Lexington, Mass.: D. C. Heath.

Gibson, J.M. (1990). National values history project. *Generations, 14:* 51–64.

Hardwig, J. (1989). In search of an ethics of personal relationships. In

G. Graham and H. LaFollette (eds.), *Person to Person,* pp. 63–81. Philadelphia: Temple University Press.

Janis, I., and Mann, L. (1977). *Decision-making: A Psychological Analysis of Conflict, Choice, and Commitment.* New York: Free Press.

Kane, R.A., and Caplan, A.L. (eds.). (1993). *Ethical Conflicts in the Management of Home Care: The Case Manager's Dilemma.* New York: Springer Publishing Co.

Kane, R.A., Penrod, J.D., and Kivnick, H.Q. (1994). Case managers discuss ethics: Dilemmas of an emerging occupation in long-term care in the United States. *Journal of Case Management,* 6: 3–12.

Kane, R.L., and Kane, R.A. (eds.). (1982). *Values and Long-Term Care.* Lexington, Mass.: D. C. Heath.

Langer, E.J. (1989). *Mindfulness.* Reading, Mass.: Addison-Wesley.

Langer, E.J., and Rodin, J. (1976). The effects of choice and enhanced personal responsibility for the aged. *Journal of Personal and Social Psychology, 34:* 191–198.

Lidz, C.W., Fischer, L., and Arnold R.M. (1992). *The Erosion of Autonomy in Long-Term Care.* New York: Oxford University Press.

Mercer, S.O., and Kane, R.A. (1979). Helplessness and hopelessness among the institutionalized elderly. *Health and Social Work,* 4: 91–116.

Morris, J.N., Hawes, C., Fries, B.E., Phillips, C.D., Mor, V., Katz, S., Murphy, K., Drugovich, M.L., and Friedlob, A. (1990). Designing the national resident assessment instrument for nursing homes. *Gerontologist,* 30: 293–307.

Quinn, J. (1993). *Successful Case Management in Long-Term Care.* New York: Springer Publishing Co.

Schulz, R. (1976). Effects of control and predictability on the physical and social well-being of the institutionalized aged. *Journal of Personal and Social Psychology, 33:* 563–573.

Seligman, M. (1975). *Helplessness: Depression, Development, and Death.* San Francisco: W. H. Freeman.

Thuras, P.D., Kane, R.A., Penrod, J.D., and Finch, M.D. (1992). Caregiver perceptions of post-hospital care decisions: Conscious or automatic? Presented at the Annual Meeting of the Gerontological Society of America, Washington, D.C.

Tobin, S.S. (1991). *Personhood in Advanced Old Age: Implications for Practice.* New York: Springer Publishing Co.

Tulloch, J. (in press, 1995). The resident's view of autonomy. In L.J. Gamroth and E. Tornquiest (eds.), *Meaningful Lives in Nursing Homes: Enhancing Resident Autonomy.* New York: Springer Publishing Co.

Tversky, A., and Kahneman, D. (1981). The framing of decisions and the psychology of choice. *Science, 211*: 453–458.

Tversky, A., Sattath, S., and Slovic, P. (1988). Contingent weighting in judgment and choice. *Psychological Review, 95*: 371–384.

Tymchuk, A.J., Ouslander, J.G., Rahbar, B., and Fitten, J. (1988). Medical decisionmaking among elderly people in long-term care. *Gerontologist, 28*: 59–63.

III RETHINKING BASIC CONCEPTS

CHAPTER SIX

Actual Autonomy and Long-Term Care Decision Making

George J. Agich

Respecting autonomy in long-term care is frequently a rather vexatious matter because the conditions that bring elders into long-term care—confusion, dementia, wandering, and a host of diseases associated with being old—are such that the very capacity for choice and rational decision making is seriously compromised, if not absent. For this reason, I have argued that the concept of autonomy in long-term care needs radical revision (Agich, 1990). It needs to be refocused on the everyday aspects of the elder's action in the social world of long-term care (Agich, 1993), as Bart Collopy also argues in this volume (Chap. 7). In the present chapter I focus on the more restricted question of the ethical dimensions of decision making in long-term care. I argue that the importance of the concept of autonomy for the ethics of long-term care is to be found more in terms of everyday decision making than the more commonly acknowledged decision making in situations of conflict or important life transitions. To elaborate this orientation within present constraints, I develop my analysis in terms of a relationship among three salient features of long-term care decision making, namely, the concept of decision making itself, the events occasioning decision making, and the operative view of autonomy. Each of these points contains a pair of distinctions that define parallel models of decision making in long-term care. I first discuss the distinctions, second, discuss the models that they compose, third, present an action-oriented view of decision making, and

Research upon which this chapter is based was supported in part by the Retirement Research Foundation.

fourth, consider some of the implications of actual autonomy for long-term care decision making.

A Framework for Discussing Autonomy in Long-Term Care
Decision Making

Decision making in long-term care can be according to either of two models, namely, nodal or interstitial. *Nodal decision making* is the term I use to refer to decision making under conditions in which clear alternatives are present, in which weighing costs and benefits is relevant, and in which coercion is possible, in part because of the disparity of power between individuals making decisions and the agencies providing care described by Terrie Wetle in Chapter 4. The decision by an elder about whether to stay at home or move to a nursing home is a nodal decision. I use the term *interstitial decision making* to refer to a class of decisions that lack the drama and discernible conflict of the former. Phenomenologically, this class of decision making includes actions that are usually not even experienced as matters of explicit decision, but rather simply as habitual ways of acting and interacting. For example, decisions are not always made, but are frequently reached. Sometimes, one comes to or arrives at a decision without the experience of having made the decision. Sometimes, the decision is evident only retrospectively. Interstitial decisions involve what is placed in one's nursing home room and the sort of decisions that shape the two cases discussed by Collopy in the next chapter.

This kind of (usually) tacit decision making points away from situations marked by interpersonal conflict over momentous matters to situations of everyday choice that reveal the ideals, beliefs, or values that are not just held or asserted in the course of disagreement, but are *personally* held and lived every day by the individual in question. A full treatment of this subject would thus need to explore the nuances of the language of decision making which, as Rosalie Kane pointed out in Chapter 5, is far more complex than might first be thought. For present purposes, it is helpful to note that the term *decision* refers not only to the act of reaching a conclusion or passing a judgment on a matter or contest but also refers to the quality of determination, firmness, or decidedness of character. This meaning of decision reminds us that the ethically most important touchstone for the analysis of long-term care involves reference to the elder who is the focus of long-term care decision making. As such, the elder is a concrete person with actual commitments, interests, and values. The decision making that occurs in the course of daily life is the most relevant, because it gives expression to the operative sense of self. The concept of interstitial decision making helps to illuminate the ethical dimensions of long-term care as a way of life, a concept discussed earlier by Nancy Wilson (Chap. 3).

Events

Parallel to this decision-making distinction is a distinction between two kinds of events or occurrences, namely, paradigm and typical. This distinction is meant to cut across a wide range of experiential phenomena including action and choice. *Paradigm events* are those that are treated as the model or exemplar of ethical conflict or dilemmas in long-term care. As such, these cases are regarded as embodying or representing rules that constitute the moral framework for long-term care. These paradigm cases are emblematic of a particular normative model of autonomy, and they reveal its special commitments. These cases involve situations in which decisions are made under conditions of adversity and conflict. The legal rights of elders to informed consent for medical treatment, for example, are readily at hand serving to protect and insulate the elder as an autonomous agent from the coercive and intrusive, even if beneficent, actions of professional caregivers or family members. In short, the paradigm events are those in which conflict or, at least, disagreement, occurs. Such cases easily engender appeal to legal rights and are typified by acute care, as discussed later in this volume by John Arras (Chap. 10) and Laurence McCullough and his colleagues (Chap. 11).

Although it is undeniable that paradigm events occur with regularity in long-term care, it is also certain that these events do not exhaust the class of ethically important problems in long-term care. Other events, though less dramatic and less amenable to definitive delineation in terms of elders' rights and providers' obligations, are at least as significant as the dramatic and conflict-ridden paradigm events. Such events comprise the vast majority of long-term care; they are the *typical events* of everyday care and social interaction that make up long-term care as Kane and Wetle illustrate in earlier chapters. Such events include performing various ADL or having them performed for oneself as well as various communicative encounters in the course of caregiving and care receiving. They are to be found not in the crises or conflicts that punctuate long-term care, but in the interstices of daily, routine action and interaction where elders live their lives and experience their world. They involve the way that care is conceived, delivered, and received; they include the inconveniences and burdens associated with the need for care and the emotional and existential problems of living with disability and frailty in the face of death.

Theory of Autonomy

Paradigm events and nodal decision making provide fertile ground for the mainstream liberal view of autonomy that dominates most contemporary bioethics theory. In this view, which is considered at greater length in Chapter 10 by Arras, to be autonomous means to be able to function as an independent, rational decision maker, as one who knows his or her own desires and preferences, and whose freedom is expressed in actions or choices that are directed at the fulfillment of desire and preference. I term this view of autonomy *ideal,* because it abstracts from the complex concrete detail that actually comprises lived (moral) experience in the world. It is intellectually seductive, because it provides a framework for analysis that admits a considerable degree of clarity and about which there is a remarkable consensus. Its applicability, however, is severely limited in long-term care insofar as the very conditions of frailty and impairment that make long-term care necessary erode the robust independence that this view of autonomy implies.[1] Nevertheless, this model is widely accepted and constitutes a kind of fulcrum in modern thinking.

Parallel to this culturally commonplace model of autonomy is a less well-known example of autonomy that is far more ordinary and widely accepted than even the former.[2] What I termed *typical events,* namely, the myriad activities and experiences of everyday life, are correlated with a different and far more pervasive, though tacit, sense of autonomy that is present as a universal background or horizon for our experience in the social world. This sense of *actual autonomy,* illustrated effectively in the two cases discussed by Collopy in Chapter 7, is less a formal model or normative theory than a characterization of the ways that autonomy is actually manifest in the social world of action. Much like a figure upon a ground, the liberal model of autonomy and the paradigm events that exemplify it stand in the forefront of our intellectual consciousness, whereas the actual manifestation of autonomy in social life comprises what is tacit and utterly taken for granted in everyday experience. Just because they are typical, these events and the autonomy revealed therein comprise the background of the quotidian world of long-term care which elders, family members, and professional care providers actually occupy.

Models of Long-Term Care Decision Making
Nodal Decision Making

The main features of nodal decision making are clearly evident in paradigm events that define the ethical dilemmas usually associated with long-term care. These paradigm events are best characterized as transitions between one stage or kind of life circumstance or life setting and another—for example, in decisions regarding institutionalization, securing in-home care, moving from intermediate to skilled nursing care, as well as decisions to commence, withhold, or withdraw various kinds of interventions ranging from in-hospital diagnostic workups for fever to surgery or other invasive treatment, such as cardiopulmonary resuscitation. These circumstances share the following characteristics. First, decision making is explicit. Choices are to be made among alternatives that are themselves perceived to be clearly demarcated. Second, there is conflict or dilemma associated with choice. Third, the options or alternatives available for choice are relatively clear. Fourth, the choice or decision making occurs under conditions of adversity. And fifth, the decisions are sometimes made in a context that is itself coercive. The standard response to these features involves reliance on a model that prizes independent free choice under conditions of a rational estimation of alternatives in light of one's personal preferences (Arras, Chap. 10).

Consider, for example, the decision whether to institutionalize an elder. In the first instance, the decision making is explicit. A choice, sometimes among alternatives, must be made, but the decision to institutionalize or not is itself decisive. Either the elder is to continue living alone with inadequate or no support or the elder is to be institutionalized for his or her own comfort or protection. The reality of the alternatives and the material costs are clearly ingredients in this kind of decision. For example, the question of payment, disposition of property, and continuity of contact with friends and family are all elements at stake. Frequently, there is a conflict or dilemma associated with this decision. The circumstances, of course, vary from case to case, but whether it is the elder, the family, or social agencies who must make the decision, there is inevitable conflict: for example, elders deciding for institutionalization in order to spare their spouses from being consumed by their care; a spouse who has to admit defeat or ineptitude in meeting the needs of a frail or demented elder spouse; or children deciding that a parent's preference for a personally comfortable and familiar, though possibly unsafe, life in familiar surroundings should be traded for a measure of protection even at the cost of what is perceived as confinement. Evidently, the options available appear all too clear.

The conflict that is experienced in the decision-making process is experienced precisely because the alternatives appear to be so well demarcated. The clarity of the alternatives is an important factor contributing to the conflictual nature of the decision to institutionalize. Because the alternatives are set out in such clear relief, the decision appears not only dramatic and momentous, but irrevocable and not subject to negotiation or revision. Although the standard analysis of institutionalization presents a clear alternative, the choice need not be binary. In many instances, elders or their families have a range of options, admittedly some more feasible than others. Besides remaining at home or moving into a nursing home, there is sometimes the possibility of in-home care, of moving in with an adult child, or of an adult child returning home to assume a caregiving role. Despite the range of choice, the alternatives are nonetheless clear, and the main conflict is presented in terms of the elder's loss of freedom, even when that loss is largely symbolic because the elder is so frail or impaired.[3] In these cases, the model supports surrogate decision making as the primary focus of ethical concern (Wetle, Chap. 4). In part, the particular sense of conflict between maintaining independence or submitting to dependence is undoubtedly shaped by the cultural attitudes and beliefs associated with institutionalization and nursing homes in our society (Goffman, 1960, 1961; Vladeck, 1980), but the element of conflict is evident in nodal decision making generally, not just the decision regarding institutionalization.

Nodal decision making is frequently conditioned by adversity. Avoidance, denial, or simply ignorance postpones decisions to the point where adversity reigns. The realization that an elder is too frail or incapacitated to remain in present surroundings frequently strikes the decision maker as an affliction or a burden. A spouse or family members will experience this realization as a calamity or hardship that cannot be reversed. Hence, the decision is usually made under circumstances of great emotional turmoil marked by an element of duress. The degree of suffering or tragedy that accompanies decision making under these conditions is readily recognized as a problem to be addressed or resolved, though the model of autonomy that is most often applied in cases of nodal decision making seems quite unsuited to deal adequately with this realization.

Finally, the decisions that are made are constrained by circumstances that are themselves frequently coercive. In part, the aforementioned sense of adversity contributes to the coercive nature of the choices at hand, but the alternatives themselves, including their economic, personal, and social costs, are also seen to threaten or influence choice. Frequently, the coercive atmosphere is personified by an individual, either a family member or as Wetle describes in Chapter 4, a professional caregiver, who presses for institutionalization of the elder. In these instances, the characteristics of nodal decision making are remarkably congruent with common understandings of the nature of autonomy in terms of which appeal to the elder's rights of self-determination and independence is readily sounded.

Nodal decision making that focuses on paradigm transition events is thus associated with a certain view of autonomy. Indeed, standard interpretations of the paradigm events of long-term care directly rely on the broadly liberal model of autonomy that so dominates contemporary bioethics. According to this model, independence is prized, and freedom of choice must be respected. Choice is to be respected, because it is the autonomous expression of the preference of the person as subject. *Autonomous expression* means both that the choice is uncoerced and that it issues from the subjective preferences of the choosing subject. The person is regarded as someone who has particular values and beliefs, enjoys a capacity for choice, and has, by his or her very nature, a fundamental right to make an uncoerced, if not unfettered, choice and to possess the objects of such a choice.

Interstitial Decision Making

The majority of day-to-day experience, however, does not conform to such a view. Decisions in everyday life belong to a different class of events. Not only are the matters of choice ordinary and routine, they are inadequately captured by a conceptual scheme dominated by conflict and rights. Certainly, everyday decisions involve (implicit) rights, claims, and sometimes conflict and disagreement, but appeals to rights describe these cases with considerably less frequency than is usually thought. This is partly true because actual autonomy is far more complexly variegated than the ideal model of autonomous choice implies. In the first instance, ideal autonomy regards individuals as fundamentally independent and isolated entities, whereas autonomy is actually exercised not by solitary individuals, but by socially situated agents engaged in interpersonal interactions. Hence, the ready appeal to forbearance that functions so effectively in the ideal model, drawn from the political/legal realm, is frequently inappropriate in the space of the family or caregiving institution.

Instead of conflictual encounters with strangers, the relationships involve shared histories and responsibility, friendship, love, or loyalty, which are considered in detail by Nancy Jecker in Chapter 8 and Sarah Brakman in Chapter 9. As a result, what is simply in "my" private interest or a matter of "my" personal preferences versus the competing interests and preferences of another is, in the usual case, more intimately intertwined and so less starkly in opposition. Even in cases in which there is conflict, it is conflict that is psychologically charged and dark with a sense of history. For this reason, decision making is not the lucid rational exercise of some calculus of preferences but is emotionally clouded. Thus, making decisions about home care is not simply a matter of deciding whose preferences, for example, the elder, family members, or professional care providers, should override all others, but more likely involves the task of coordinating and subordinating various interests and preferences, many of which are shared, and the task of discovering and accommodating various attitudes, beliefs, and feelings, some of which are more nebulous than clear.

The ethical importance of autonomy for long-term care is to be found more in the overwhelmingly rich character of everyday life and experience than in the liminal cases of conflict which exist on the fringes of long-term care. So regarded, the problem that autonomy poses cannot be the straightforward—at least theoretically straightforward—problem of addressing the conditions that coerce choice or constrain the free exercise of preference that is so well expressed in standard ethical analysis. Such conditions are, after all, in principle not eliminable for any finite being and are even harder to overlook in the case of elders who require long-term care.

Actual autonomy thus focuses less on the freedom of choice than it does on the concrete reality of the one who chooses. Actual autonomy is, however, never just a matter of choice under hypothesized conditions; instead, it is manifested in the myriad actions that comprise one's everyday existence. Autonomy is thus revealed less in deliberate reflective choice than in everyday actions undertaken on the basis of habit and disposition. Habit and disposition manifest the autonomy of the agent in an automatic fashion, that is, without the critical reflective distance that standard accounts of ideal autonomy require.[4] Instead, the task involves understanding and respecting who the elder is as an actual agent in the world. To do so is far less a matter of assuring that elders' choices are respected than it is to know whether the choices afforded frail and disabled elders accord with who they fundamentally are. The most important examples of interstitial decision making for the ethics of long-term care involve situations that are not usually regarded as decisions, because they are made habitually or routinely in the course of quotidian life.

Autonomy literally means "self-rule," that is, behavior that is spontaneous and self-initiated; such behavior is regarded as action in the sense that it manifests intentionality. Human action, in turn, can be regarded as free if the individual agent can identify with the elements from which it flows; an action (or choice) is unfree or coerced if the agent cannot identify with or dissociates from the elements that generate or prompt the action (Bergmann, 1977, p. 37). This means that the ability to identify with the constituents of an action is logically prior to freedom. Actual autonomy is founded on the possession of a formed identity or of a self having a particular determinate nature and character. Expressions of autonomy are thus the enactments of who the individual is in the social world of everyday life. Such enactments are not confined to the realm of deliberative choice but find expression in clothing, dietary, or entertainment preferences, or in habitual ways of speaking and turning a phrase. All of these commonplace behaviors reveal who the elder is. Because identification is socially situated, caregiving practices in nursing homes or home care can either support the development and exercise of the concrete autonomy of the unique person or thwart or stunt the expression of the self (Bergmann, 1977, p. 39).[5] Action is an engagement in the ambient world. It is embodied choice as illustrated by Mrs. Marner and Mr. Rand in Collopy's case studies in the next chapter. Actual autonomy is not well served by standardized, "cookie cutter" care plans against which Kane cautioned in the previous chapter.

Autonomous action and choice thus reflect, create, and sustain character, disposition, and habit. The traditional conception of autonomy as rational, free agency implies that free actions are the result of a reflective, deliberative process that yields a decision defensible on rational grounds. With this view, prior reflection and decision are necessary for an action to be judged as free. This condition establishes an unrealistically and unremittingly high standard for autonomy in long-term care—and everyday life in general as well.

For real persons, autonomy always involves developed patterns. I am autonomous because my thoughts move *automatically* through my fingers and into my computer not less. The skill or habit of typing enhances and extends my autonomy rather than limits it. The relationship between what is done automatically in normal human experience and autonomy unfortunately has been effaced because attention has been constricted to the phenomena associated with choice and will in most philosophical treatments. In a fuller sense, specific actions or choices can be judged to be truly free or unfree not simply because the agent did perform some particular deliberative or reflective validation, but to the extent that they are consistent with the elder's self-identity.

In standard views, everyday actions or choices that are habitual or taken for granted are either uninteresting or seem unfree. Such actions and choices, however, are animated by a self-awareness that is an essential feature of consciousness. In terms of actual autonomy, however, such actions and choices are truly free or unfree to the extent that they are consistent with the person's self-identify. The requirement that explicit rational decision making underlies all truly free action or choice is an idealization that makes sense only in light of an abstract or idealized view of the self. Actual persons, however, could not long endure the burden of analysis and deliberation that such a view implies.

Actual autonomy, in short, is an engaged and preoccupied autonomy. It is thus more important to think of autonomy in long-term care in terms of who the elder actually is and with what things the elder in fact identifies than ideal conditions of free choice. One can, after all, clearly respect the conditions of free choice by affording options that themselves violate the integrity of the elder as a developed person. For this reason, identification precedes the concept of freedom and provides a foundation for any truly practical treatment of autonomy in long-term care.

An Action-Oriented View of Decision Making

Ethnographic research in nursing homes has demonstrated a remarkably bureaucratic and medical environment that is more institutional than home-like (Gubrium, 1975; Lidz, Fischer, and Arnold, 1992; Savishinsky, 1991; Shield, 1988). The most basic requisites for a home, such as the sense of personal or personalized space, control of time, and privacy, are seldom found in nursing homes, yet the elder is expected to "reside" therein. Clearly, these are contradictory expectations that introduce stressful complications into nursing home care. Because the elder is not displaced, home care is assumed by many to be more desirable. Unfortunately, the houses in which elders are left after the departure of children and the loss of a spouse or of their own capacity for self-care can be symbolically transformed into a place of strangeness. Alienation from family and friends may originate in or be exacerbated by a primal sense of alienation from one's everyday surroundings. The common view that institutionalization inevitably brings to the frail elder a fundamental sense of loss may only be superficially true. Rather, a house full of memories and ghosts might be even more unhomelike at a deeper level.

Whether the locus of care is an institution or one's own home, all persons need a sense of place wherein one feels comfortable or at one with oneself. In part, this sense seems rooted in a physical place but is actually moveable; it originates with the privileged space of one's own body and the primary developmental space in which the self emerged. The lived body is the locus of embodied action through which the person reveals and discovers herself in the world in interaction with others. The frailties and incapacities associated with old age, however, introduce fractures into this primal organ of being in the world that distort the lived body's expressive functionality. With the experience of such fractures, the elder naturally feels vulnerable and engages in various adaptive strategies. Interpreting the actions of elders in long-term care as simply ineffective and irrational or as symptoms of a (usually ill-determined) disease process effectively cuts off the prospect of seeing the elder's autonomy actually manifest in the elder's life, a theme also explored in the next chapter by Collopy. When the experience of illness and debility, memory loss, and physical incapacity are filtered through an interpretative environment that marginalizes adaptive efforts, the actual autonomy of the elder is effectively thwarted. It is thwarted not at center stage in a dramatic fashion rife with conflict and spiced by appeal to rights, but off-stage in the myriad caregiving interactions that comprise the daily world of long-term care. The autonomy actually manifested by frail and incapacitated elders is understandably preoccupied with adaptive effort. Alterations in the elder's physical surroundings and basic sense of space, thus, can either compound or serve to ameliorate these experiences. Under these circumstances, it is essential that the elder be regarded as an agent struggling to adapt or readjust to altered surroundings. Viewing the elder's effort as adaptive moves one away from the abstract, rational decision model so frequently used toward a more realistic and practically useful approach, an approach that focuses on the particular meanings and significance of the environment for the elder trying to adapt with compromised capacities.

To focus on adaptive effort entails that the elder is first viewed concretely as a formed self. Given that the majority of elders in nursing homes are without family or others who know the elder well, attaining this kind of understanding might seem impossible. However, the concept of actual autonomy provides a ready access. What is needed is not a comprehensive history but an opportunity to participate in the narrative unfolding of elders' present efforts against the background of their character, dispositions, and habits. Instead of an attention to past medical and social history, it might be better to focus efforts on understanding the elder's present experiences by allowing actual caregiving staff appropriate opportunities for meaningful interactions, as Collopy suggests in the next chapter. Elders' stories are, of course, still important, but not as insights into the nature of the person as preformed but as expressions of the kind of people the elders were and want to be, the kinds of beliefs and values that they personally hold. As such, an elder's life story not only needs opportunities for being told and being heard, but also opportunities for retelling and reworking as the daily experiences of long-term care take their place in the actual life of the elder.

One primary task for caregivers should be to foster the efforts of elders to reorient themselves by active cooperation in the elders' efforts to remake their world. The process of world making (and remaking) is an important but often overlooked aspect of adaptation to loss, pain, and suffering (Scarry, 1985). Remaking the world cannot, however, occur generically. No rule can be reliably followed nor given to another. Instead, elders must try in their own unique way to constitute a personal world through various interpretive efforts. The effective and ethically responsive caregiver will have to be open to an interpretive understanding of this process if actual autonomy is to be respected. This effort, it needs to be stressed, is *effort*; it involves work. It is primarily an effort of the elder in which the caregiver may be privileged to participate or witness. In this regard, a number of preconceptions about elders in long-term care must be critically reassessed.

Frail and dependent elders are not just passive recipients of someone else's acts—even institutionalized elders regularly reveal activity if we are prepared to recognize it. Unfortunately, institutionalized elders are defined by the social structure and organization of nursing homes in a passive way. They are named in terms of their diseases and their basic record of care, the chart, which primarily concerns what is done to them, such as feeding, bathing, or toileting, not what they do. To outside observers it might appear to be a passive existence; infrequent short visits provide snapshot images of people "just sitting" (Diamond, 1986, p. 1289). To be sure, day rooms filled with a score of elders are typically bereft of conversation or other apparently meaningful interactions. There is, however, another side to the surface reality of life in a nursing home that evades most casual observers; this reality extends beyond these static images to reveal the operation of agency. Once one gets to know elders as individuals, it becomes clear that almost all are thinking and conscious people, though their consciousness might be fragile and intermittent and their concerns different from our own.

The same is true of elders residing in their own homes. To caregivers, especially family members, the frail elder might appear withdrawn or uninterested in aspects of the home or activities that occurred therein previously. It would be a mistake to assume that such instances of disengagement represent a passivity on the part of the elder; rather, such elders may struggle to accept limitations on activities and might grieve over their inability to carry out personally meaningful or significant functions. Such reactions deserve careful and individually attuned responses. Other elders might compensate for their reduced capacities by demanding that others perform what might seem to be empty ritual functions, such as decorating the home for Halloween, Christmas, or other holidays or doing spring cleaning. Reasoning that the elder has no children at home or no grandchildren near to warrant the Halloween planning, that the Christmas dinner would be better held at a child's home, or that the house hasn't seen enough activity during the winter to warrant a full-scale house cleaning might completely miss the mark. In the absence of a sensitive awareness of the various meanings, including the symbolic meaning, of these activities for the elder, caregivers can all too easily overlook how their own acceptance or rejection of the background beliefs and values associated with these practices might complicate how these matters are handled. Simply insisting either on the elder's or the caregiver's right to exercise free choice about such matters is singularly unhelpful. However, because actual autonomy acknowledges the psychological and social situation of individuals, it makes possible an understanding of the complex processes of interpretation and negotiation that are at work in these kinds of decision making.

In reality elders are not simply acted upon but struggle to maintain their own consciousness and identity, even if appearances sometimes belie this effort (Diamond, 1986, pp. 1289–1290). Appearances belie this effort because we assume that real work is objectified in the world as a "work," a material object produced by one's efforts. Work, however, is actually closely related to the phenomena of pain and imagination; like them it presses toward objectification, though the objectification is not always so evidently a physical thing in the world (Scarry, 1985). Rather, the work activities in which many (particularly institutionalized) elders engage involve reconstituting the meaning structures of their lives, not simply forming objects within the ambient world. Too often the kind of interpretive effort required for such world making is overlooked, because standard accounts of autonomy never adequately address the need for individuals to actively make a world, focusing instead on discrete choices or decisions within a pregiven frame of reference.

Actual autonomy thus requires that the routine and ordinary actions of elders be understood as a fundamentally creative engagement in and interaction with their environment. Actual autonomy also highlights the participatory role that caregivers need to undertake. Instead of thinking of the elder simply as an array of symptoms or aberrant behaviors that need management, caregivers must think of the elder as one who is actively engaged in world making. Because interstitial decision making occurs in the midst of daily life, attention must be given to the social and personal meanings of routine caregiving interactions with elders and less to the bureaucratic bed and body work described by Jaber Gubrium (1975, pp. 123–157). The home-care analog of bed and body work are those activities designed to accomplish specific objective and measurable results for the elder without necessarily integrating the elder's personal sense of purpose, timing, or value.

Some Implications of Actual Decision Making

Focusing on actual autonomy has a wide range of implications for long term care decision making. Two examples can be used to demonstrate this range: the issue of restraints and the problem of dependence.

Movement and the Significance of Space

The issue of the use of physical restraints on elders in long-term care needs to be placed in the wider context of the meaning of movement and space for actual autonomy. The concept of actual autonomy is meant to highlight the complex circumstance that I have called the mundane experience of long-term care. That experience is composed of a variegated pattern of actions and interactions in which elders, like all social agents, engage. These activities occur on the basis of "sedimented" experiences recognized as character traits, dispositions, or habits. These sedimented experiences also include a vast store of recipes for action composing a stock of knowledge at hand that plays a crucial role in any understanding or analysis of everyday experience. Sociologists refer to these structures of experiences as "typifications" and stress the way that typifications order experience by establishing patterned expectations and by providing frameworks of relevance.[6] Frail and disabled elders who require long-term care experience their world in a similar manner but with the added complication that their experiences are mediated by memory or perceptual deficits, pain, and disabilities, such as mobility limitation. Some elders, especially those suffering cognitive or memory impairments, manifest confusion and exhibit wandering. These behaviors, because of their potential for physical harm, have led caregivers to adopt restrictive attitudes toward such elders.

For example, nursing homes frequently report that they are forced to restrain these elders for fear of lawsuit. However, as of 1989 no lawsuit had been successful against a facility solely for failure to restrain a resident. In fact, the risk of liability for false imprisonment, assault, or injury or death from restraint is much greater with misuse of physical restraints (Blakeslee, Goldman, and Papougenis, 1990, p. 80).[7] To replace physical restraints, however, requires not only adopting an individualized approach to care, but also a recognition that these elders are capable, despite their frailties, of a potential for meaningful expressions of autonomy. The recognition is counterintuitive for many who think that the only definitive examples of autonomy are cases of rational decision making, despite the fact that human decision making hardly conforms to this ideal. These beliefs about the rational nature of decision making not only complicate the problem of wandering but permeate the whole subject of long-term care decision making and are a source of the ethical challenges to case managers discussed earlier by Kane (Chap. 5) and Wetle (Chap. 4).

Respecting the elder's need for freedom of movement is not just a matter of trading off safety for independence, because these concerns are much more closely related than is usually thought. As Collopy argues in the next chapter, a concern for safety that is defined narrowly in physical or medical terms tends to ignore broad classes of other important harms, such as social or psychological harms. The concept of actual autonomy helps us to understand why this is so. The key to a restraint-free approach to the care of the wandering and confused elders thus involves a conceptual change on the part of caregivers. Staff are required to depart from normal bed and body work and actively work toward resolving the particular problem by attempting to understand the meaning latent in the seemingly purposeless movement of the cognitively impaired elder. Maintaining mobility and independence involves more than simply assuring safety and security but consists as well in eliminating environmental barriers in order to provide opportunities for meaningful wandering.[8] If wandering is not viewed as a problem to be controlled but as an opportunity to engage individuals in actions that occur along well-defined, secure, and engaging paths, then wandering behavior of the cognitively impaired elder can permit mobility and independence to occur (Cohen and Weisman, 1990, p. 76; Cohen and Weisman, 1991).

Because the spatial environment is such an important facet of actual autonomy, its use to either control elders or enhance their choice and range of experience is an important aspect in respecting the actual autonomy of elders in long-term care. Electing protection without considering the costs to the quality of experience of the cognitively impaired elder is to thwart rather than respect the elder's autonomy. Coons (1987) suggested that rigid schedules and hospital-like design elements are not suitable for long-term care, particularly for residents who are cognitively impaired. What is needed is an environment that affords opportunities to express developed tendencies and habits by affording a variety of spaces ranging from private to public. Such choice facilitates elders' control of both their sensory and social stimulation and may reduce the perceived intrusion or threat to their own individual space. The operative sense of identification, understood as the rudiment of freedom, provides a positive and practical ground for enhancing a range of meaningful choices for the confused and cognitively impaired elder. As Cohen and Weisman put it:

> To the extent that individuals have the opportunity to make meaningful decisions about their environments, they can maintain ties to their past lives. ... For people with dementia, familiar artifacts, activities, and spaces can provide valuable personal associations and can stimulate opportunities for

social interaction and meaningful activity. Rather than being limited to a single "rummage box," the total environment may be utilized to trigger reminiscence. (Cohen and Weisman, 1990, p. 76.)

Dependence and Actual Autonomy

Elders who require in-home or institutional care are dependent in important ways. The nodal decision making model implies that it is a primary ethical requirement that elders be accorded freedom of choice. Such an approach, however, can readily overlook the fact that a person can be free to choose but unable to enact the choice. Decisional autonomy does not always imply executional ability, especially for frail or incapacitated elders (Collopy, 1988). Viewed interstitially decision making is located in everyday actions that reveal and enact dispositions and habits. If actual autonomy and not some disembodied ideal is to be taken seriously, then decision making cannot be restricted to assuring noncoercive conditions but must attend as well to the conditions that enhance elders' practical capacities to express their developed sense of self. Nonetheless, some elders are clearly able to choose in line with ideal autonomy yet lack the functional abilities to enact their choices. For these cases respecting autonomy is more a matter of providing appropriate means for elders to exercise their choices. In other instances, the executional incapacity is coincident with a decisional incapacity. These latter cases present the most interesting challenge for any theory of autonomy in long-term care.

The standard response to cases of decisional incapacity, of course, involves an appeal to a surrogate decision making. This response follows naturally from the model of ideal autonomy and serves its limited purposes. The problem is that these purposes are restricted to decisional crises and so cannot readily be extended widely in long-term care. Surrogate decision making simply substitutes another decision maker for the incompetent elder with the view that the exercise of autonomy can be readily transferred from one unable to meet the ideal conditions of rational and free choice to others who can. This preserves the primacy of autonomy for decision making but does so on an extremely abstract plane. Although surrogate decision making is understandable, and perhaps even defensible as a legal fiction created to solve certain critical clinical ethical problems, it can displace other vital ethical considerations. It is especially troublesome in long-term care, insofar as it does not help to disclose the everyday reality of long-term care. In fact, it leads caregivers in the wrong direction by setting out an unattainably high standard. Not finding frail and incapacitated elders to be rational, free, independent agents, caregivers are encouraged to overlook the elders' actual manifestations of autonomy in their daily caregiving encounters!

Choice, like action, is inevitable for humans. The issue concerns the definition and meaning of choice (and action) for severely compromised elders. Actual autonomy, by focusing on interstitial decision making, views decisions as an essential feature of the social life of elders in long-term care. Thus, by definition elders who are capable of any kind of interaction with caregivers or of merely responding to caregiving demonstrate at least the minimal degree of agency necessary for actual autonomy. This minimal agency, however, is intertwined with the elder's dependence and so might easily be overlooked. Identifying and supporting the elder's dispositions and habits as they are exhibited in the course of routine caregiving interactions may seem to be more a matter of effective caregiving than respect for autonomy, unless we realize that an appropriately sensitive response to a dependent other is grounded in the recognition of that other as a unique person or individual. This sense of a person is not an abstraction but is experientially present to caregivers in the elder's reactions to the caregiving; it is expressed in the likes or dislikes that are manifested in the course of everyday care. Such likes and dislikes reveal the habits and traits that actually comprise who the individual is. Taking note of these tendencies and respecting them is thus one way to respect actual autonomy of elders who lack decisional capacity.

Illness, including loss of cognitive, physical, or social function, invariably involves a dissolution of the primordial unity of the self, the body, and the world. Normally in the everyday world the self is experienced as one with one's action. The body is simply the vehicle for achieving ends in the world and is transparent to our intentions. Illness heralds the need to depend on others to compensate for one's shortcomings. This dependence is expressed in the very social world of the elder. It includes needing help in performing ADL. The ill or incapacitated elder is dependent, sometimes pervasively so, on others in a way that is atypical for most adults. This situation leads either to experiences of hope and trust, for example, as spousal (Jecker, Chap. 8) or filial responsibility (Brakman, Chap. 9) comes into play or new responsibility relationships develop, or despair and mistrust as the sick elder has to accommodate not only to the dependence associated with the incapacity but also to the need to rely on perfunctory caregiving (cf. Bergsma and Thomasma, 1982, p. 177).

The dependence of frail or incapacitated elders can involve a specific infantilization as the elders find themselves needful of supervision and help with basic self-care activities. In a variety of ways they are placed in the hands of others. As a result the experience of the world is refracted through the kind of care that others are willing and able to extend and also structured by the degree and kind of care that the sick elder is characteristically willing or able to accept. This latter point is important, because we sometimes think that the diagnosis determines in an objective fashion the degree or kind of help that should be offered by others. In point of fact, however, there is no objective measure of the seriousness of an illness. By definition, illness is a subjectively experienced phenomenon, and it is experienced by elders and manifested in their social world through adaptive effort; so, too, the style of care needs a degree of individual tailoring. That is probably why most elders, and people in general, prefer care rendered by those with whom they share bonds of affection, rather than strangers, no matter how well trained or qualified they may be. It is indeed ironic that so much effort is expended in trying to eliminate affect from the professional caregiving or treatment relationship (Roth, 1973), when harnessing the positive affect could help avoid the job and career routinization that is readily reported, for example, by nurse's aides (Diamond, 1986). It is often forgotten by caregivers that the attention that dependent elders give to bodily processes is necessarily part of the interpretive effort of elders trying to make sense of a fractured world that is reduced to or focused on the body and its incapacity (Bergsma and Thomasma, 1982, p. 180).

Intimacy thus naturally emerges in day-to-day caregiving. *Intimacy* refers not simply to familiarity or to affection in the caregiving relationship but to a closeness or proximity of the caregiver to the dependent elder. It is far easier in a relation of dependence for the caregiver to simply take over the care of the elder without ever intending to return it to the elder. What prevents this ordinary erosion of elders' everyday autonomy is not surrogate decision making, but a caring and respectful attitude toward elders that manifests itself in a responsibility relationship animated by the commitment to help elders maintain their identity despite the ravages of impairment.

The profound nature of dependence for elders who are both decisionally and executionally incompetent helps us to understand why autonomy seems such an alien concept in long-term care. Standard treatments import a model that is incongruent with everyday reality. In actuality, autonomy is a relevant ethical concern not just because frail elders have their freedom limited or taken away by powerful caregivers or impersonal institutional forces, but because the existential conditions that are the prerequisites for long-term care themselves make being a person a routine everyday challenge.

In the daily course of living, the question "Who am I?" is typically suspended or set aside as a conscious matter for inquiry, but that does not mean that the matter is ever really closed. The Socratic aphorism that an unexamined life is not worth living should not be taken as if philosophical reflection or psychological introspection is the only way in which such questions are explicitly opened and enjoined. Existential crises or life transitions, which include by definition long-term care decisions, are widely recognized events that prompt questions such as "Who am I?" or "In what do I believe?" Sickness, too, frequently forces an examination of what is so commonly termed one's "values." In point of fact, however, in normal daily life we are able to proceed quite nicely oblivious to our own spontaneity and freedom despite regular adjustments of intentionality as our efforts are fulfilled or frustrated in the world of actual experience. Lack of explicit reflective awareness or the cognitive ability to discuss such awareness, then, cannot be taken to imply that autonomy is not present; rather, the actual rarity of fully rational, reflective deliberation regarding courses of action and outcomes should serve to remind us that standard models of autonomy are remarkably idealized. The failure of much current ethical theory to take this point seriously seems an example of what Alfred North Whitehead termed the "fallacy of misplaced concreteness," namely, the error of mistaking the abstract for the concrete (Whitehead, 1948, p. 52).

Self-identity is not something that one discovers as an uncharted island in the middle of a sea but rather is something that is made by individuals in the very course of their living. To speak meaningfully of the autonomy of dependent elders requires that we pay attention to the kinds of things with which they identify in their lives. Saying this is to expand on the slogan "respect for persons" in a way that reflects the concrete reality of human existence. The demand that autonomy be respected takes the form of an insistence on total independence only for those individuals who truly lack identity or for those things with which individuals cannot sensibly identify (Bergmann, 1977, p. 48). If I am in harmony with something, if in fact it is me—and that is the point of talking about identification—then I need not be protected or made independent from it in order to be autonomous.[9] In the most typical circumstances of long-term care, it is quite unnecessary to dwell on such an extreme version of autonomy.

Conclusion

Like the warp of a fabric, the concept of autonomy binds various threads of our personal and social lives. But like the warp of a cloth, autonomy is not the whole of the fabric, only a constituent piece. Its presence and importance in modern thinking is undeniable; advocates and devotees of postmodernism have yet to demonstrate its dispensability. Nevertheless, the concept of autonomy is fraught with difficulties and tensions. In the context of long-term care, it focuses attention on certain kinds of problems and away from other features that are ethically important. In this paper I have discussed the way that actual autonomy is related to a strain of quite ordinary decision making in long-term care. I argued that the problem with focusing on the paradigm transition event as a model for long-term care ethics is that it emphasizes the unusual at the expense of the mundane and ordinary. The significance of the typical and everyday kind of choice and action is that it brings the ethical relevance of actual autonomy into the heart of long-term care by promoting a reexamination of a range of problems such as the use of restraints and dependence.

NOTES

1. This is actually one reason among many that restrict its broad applicability as a regulative ideal for long term care. Others include the fact that long-term care does not primarily consist of medical interventions that usually require informed consent but involves assistance with various ADL. Also, unlike acute care, long-term care is not an interlude in the course of normal life but is itself a way of life for the frail or debilitated elder.

2. This claim will seem paradoxical in light of the earlier claim that the liberal view of autonomy is itself culturally dominant and, thus, common. The paradox dissolves as soon as we recognize that the liberal model of autonomy is common precisely in virtue of its *focal* presence in our discourse about matters of ethics and law.

3. The loss of freedom that comes with long-term care is symbolic in those cases in which the incapacity is so great that it effectively erodes the elder's free-

dom. The help even more than the need that calls it forth symbolizes that free-dom is thrown off. The tendency to deny need and to hate the help represents a kind of secondary defense against dependence; it reflects a cultural attitude that has been termed *counterdependence* and is based on the assumption that inde-pendence or negative freedom is all that one can meaningfully say about auton-omy (Christiansen, 1983, pp. 52–128).

4. These remarks summarize a rather difficult issue about the nature and function of critical reflection in autonomy, namely, the status of autonomy in a split-level account of the self. (For a summary of this issue, see Friedman, 1986.)

5. It might seem odd at first glance to speak of development in the context of the characteristic loss of capacities associated with old age, but a proper un-derstanding of autonomy does reveal a sense in which one can speak of depen-dent elders as exhibiting development as they engage in adaptive effort. (See Agich, 1993, pp. 85–90.)

6. For example, on entering a room, one typically expects certain structural elements to be present, such as a ceiling. On entering a dining room in a home, one expects to find a table and chairs. These general expectations are, in actual experience, further determined, so that on entering my office, for example, I typ-ically expect not only familiar structural elements and furnishings, but that my office will be "available" to me. Availability is a concept that refers to the past uses of the office, to the artifacts contained therein—for example, my books, papers, software disks, computer, writing implements—which are not only present but meaningfully present for me as components of various projects in which I am engaged, reflecting various interests of mine, and representing various tasks to be accomplished. These expectations are thus grounded in an experienced sense of meaning that the room itself exudes for me, but not so for others. The way I identify with my office is thus not only bound up with typical expectations about its physical contents but also with various meanings and expectations associated with my personal projects, purposes, or tasks at hand. Associated with these are various experiences of anticipation, anxiety, burden, and pleasure. These elements comprise that remarkably complex, yet routinely unnoticed, world of everyday experience.

7. The use of restraints actually requires more staff than less because immo-bilization causes chronic constipation, pressure sores, loss of bone mass, muscle atrophy, decreased ability to ambulate, and eventual invalidism (Miller, 1975; Warshaw et al., 1982), so one common rationale for the use of restraints is not supported by data. In fact, studies of two communities that do not use any kind of physical restraints indicate that they have no more injuries from falls than do

facilities that employ such devices (Blakeslee, Goldman, and Papougenis, 1990, p. 80).

8. The use of alarms on the doors of the elder's room and exit doors, placement of yellow barrier strips fastened by Velcro, or use of a mat at the threshold of a doorway help deter some confused patients from entering or leaving areas. They do so by providing perceptual cues that afford elders choices to proceed or alter their movement. More staff are not necessarily required to accord elders this kind of freedom of movement, rather a commitment to one-on-one staff supervision during times when an elder is particularly anxious is necessary. Such flexibility on the part of staff members is, unfortunately, rare in the bureaucratized nursing home.

9. The idea that autonomy involves identification and the possession of a self-identity is quite evident in Mill's classic treatment of liberty. He, too, insisted that individuals require a unique and distinctive condition for their existence (Mill, 1978, pp. 64 and 65).

REFERENCES

Agich, G.J. (1990). Reassessing autonomy in long-term care. *Hastings Center Report, 20*: 12–17.

Agich, G.J. (1993). *Autonomy and Long-Term Care.* New York: Oxford University Press.

Bergmann, F. (1977). *On Being Free.* Notre Dame, Ind.: University of Notre Dame Press.

Bergsma, J., and Thomasma, D. (1982). *Health Care: Its Psychosocial Dimensions.* Pittsburgh: Duquesne University Press.

Blakeslee, J., Goldman, B., and Papougenis, D. (1990). Untying the elderly: Kendal's restraint-free program at Longwood and Crosslands. *Generations, 14*(Supplement): 79–80.

Christiansen, A.J. (1983). *Autonomy and Dependence in Old Age: An Ethical Analysis.* Yale University Doctoral Dissertation. Ann Arbor, Mich.: University Microfilms.

Cohen, U., and Weisman, G.D. (1990). Environmental design to maximize autonomy for older adults with cognitive impairments. *Generations, 14*(Supplement): 75–78.

Cohen, U., and Weisman, G.D. (1991). *Holding onto Home: Designing Environments for People with Dementia.* Baltimore: Johns Hopkins University Press.

Collopy, B.J. (1988). Autonomy and long-term care: Some crucial distinctions. *Gerontologist, 28*(Supplement): 10–17.

Coons, D. (1987). *Designing a Residential Care Unit for Persons with Dementia*. Washington, D.C.: Office of Technology Assessment.

Diamond, T. (1986). Social policy and everyday life in nursing homes: A critical ethnography. *Social Science and Medicine, 23*: 1287–1295.

Friedman, M.A. (1986). Autonomy and the split-level self. *Southern Journal of Philosophy, 24*: 19–35.

Goffman, E. (1960). Characteristics of total institutions. In M.R. Stein, A.J. Vidich, and D.M. White (eds.), *Identity and Anxiety: Survival of the Person in Mass Society*, pp. 449–479. New York: Free Press.

Goffman, E. (1961). *Asylums: Essays on the Social Situation of Mental Patients and Other Inmates*. New York: Doubleday.

Gubrium, J.F. (1975). *Living and Dying at Murray Manor*. New York: St. Martin's Press.

Lidz, C.W., Fischer, L., and Arnold, R.M. (1992). *The Erosion of Autonomy in Long-Term Care*. New York: Oxford University Press.

Mill, J.S. (1978). *On Liberty*. Indianapolis: Hackett Publishing Co.

Miller, M. (1975). Iatrogenic and nurisgenic effects of prolonged immobilization of the ill aged. *Journal of the American Geriatrics Society, 23*: 360–369.

Roth, J.R. (1973). Care of the sick: Professionalization vs. love. *Science, Medicine and Man, 1*: 173–180.

Savishinsky, J.S. (1991). *The Ends of Time: Life and Work in a Nursing Home*. New York: Bergin & Garvey.

Scarry, E. (1985). *The Body in Pain: The Making and Unmaking of the World*. New York: Oxford University Press.

Shield, R.R. (1988). *Uneasy Endings: Daily Life in an American Nursing Home*. Ithaca, N.Y.: Cornell University Press.

Vladeck, B.C. (1980). *Unloving Care: The Nursing Home Tragedy*. New York: Basic Books.

Warshaw, G.A., Moore, J.T., Friedman, S.W., Currie, C.T., Kennie, D.C., Kane, W.J., and Mears, P.A. (1982). Functional disability in the hospitalized elderly. *Journal of the American Medical Association, 248*: 847–850.

Whitehead, A.N. (1948). *Science and the Modern World*. New York: Mentor Books.

CHAPTER SEVEN

Safety and Independence:
Rethinking Some Basic Concepts in Long-Term Care

Bart J. Collopy

The Clash of Safety and Independence

In both institutional and community-based long-term care, concerns about the safety of the frail elderly often clash with concerns about their independence. As both Terrie Wetle (Chap. 4) and Rosalie Kane (Chap. 5) indicated in their earlier discussions of care planning and case management, such clashes are generally resolved in favor of safety. This suggests that, for all the recent attention given to the autonomy of patients, long-term care continues to take a highly protective stance toward the frail elderly—and a highly cautious stance toward the risks that come with their self-determination.

From an historical perspective this is no surprise. In Chapter 2 Martha Holstein and Thomas Cole described the grimly custodial almshouses that were the predecessors of modern long-term care. Twentieth-century reforms brought an end to these institutions chiefly by medicalizing long-term care and bringing dramatic improvement in modes of treatment, professional standards, public image, and government funding (Wilson, Chap. 3). But with these advances came a deep dependence on the medical model of care, a dependence that has kept long-term care ethics in tutelage to acute care ethics.

As a result, questions about the independence of nursing home residents or home care clients are still framed within the logic and ethics of *medical* decision making (Arras, Chap. 10), in terms of what George Agich termed ideal autonomy in the previous chapter. Thus, independence means autonomy, and autonomy means determining one's own medical treatment. Other areas of human independence do not figure conspicuously in the medical model. Indeed, in the hospital these other areas of independence are routinely curtailed for the sake of immediate medical goals and regimens. In the same fashion, safety also becomes a limited issue, an important value certainly, a presumed condition of the caregiving environment, but hardly a focal point in patient or provider decision making about medical treatment. Even decisions about life-sustaining care are not framed as choices between safe and unsafe care. The patient who chooses palliative over aggressive care is not left "unsafe." In fact, the very language of safety rings oddly here, as if talk relevant to building and equipment standards had intruded into the discourse of clinical ethics.

In long-term care, on the other hand, safety *is* part of the moral vernacular. The extended course of care and its "daily life" aspects do not allow the tight controls that operate in the short-term, episodic world of acute care. When care is provided for long periods of time, within a *living* as well as *treatment* setting, issues of independence reach far beyond the bounds of medical treatment decisions. Moreover, for the elderly the complications of frailty often seed independence with risk. Thus safety becomes an ubiquitous issue—and an especially conflictive one, as the following two cases illustrate. (The names used are fictitious.)

Two Illustrative Cases

CASE I

Mrs. Marner is an 83-year-old widow, living alone in a small one-bedroom apartment. Until recently her chief medical complaints were arthritis and high blood pressure, but a year ago she fell and broke her hip. After hospitalization, she returned to her apartment and recuperated there with the help of home care services. She now receives fifteen hours per week of assistance from a home care aide and monthly visits from a nurse.

Mrs. Marner's apartment is cluttered with old furniture, piles of newspapers and magazines, collapsing cardboard boxes filled with the belongings of her dead sister. Three cats roam this dusty terrain, their feeding dishes and litter boxes scattered about. The apartment has poorly working appliances. It is hot and airless in summer, poorly heated in winter, often without hot water in any season. Mrs. Marner, fearful of being robbed, rarely ventures outside the apartment. She spends her days sitting quietly in the semidark, "rummaging through the past," as she puts it.

The aide originally assigned by the home care agency found these working conditions intolerable and quickly asked to be removed from the case.

Her replacement is uneasy about the neighborhood and complains that she cannot clean the apartment decently, because Mrs. Marner will not let her move anything. The aide also has problems with Charley, Mrs. Marner's 60-year-old nephew, who is a regular and irksome visitor. Charley complains about the aide's work and gets his aunt to have the aide prepare food that *he* then eats. Ostensibly, he is Mrs. Marner's family caregiver, but as the aide sees it, he just comes around looking for free meals and money. The aide reports that Charley makes out checks that Mrs. Marner signs without reading. According to the aide, Charley "takes his percentage." By month's end, Mrs. Marner is usually low on funds, sometimes reduced to little more than soup and bread. At this point, Charley disappears until next month's social security and pension checks arrive for his aunt.

The nurse who oversees Mrs. Marner's case is concerned about all of this. She is particularly bothered by what she sees as a slide in Mrs. Marner's functional status. In the last six months her arthritis has worsened, and her mobility decreased measurably. Her short-term memory also seems to be failing, and she often forgets to take her blood pressure medication. In general, her earlier self-caring and self-directing capacities have slipped noticeably.

During her monthly visit with Mrs. Marner the nurse suggests that the agency increase the hours of assistance Mrs. Marner receives. And she raises with Mrs. Marner the prospect of nursing home placement. Mrs. Marner abruptly rejects both suggestions. The aide is helpful and friendly enough, Mrs. Marner says, but she likes her privacy, and, besides, the aide doesn't get along with Charley. The nursing home is simply out of the question. "I want to stay in my own place. I've been here for thirty-five years. A nursing home is no place to be."

CASE 2

Mr. Rand is a 78-year-old nursing home resident, a diabetic with Parkinson's disease. He has been in the nursing home for six months and during that time has become an increasingly "problematic" resident in the eyes of the staff. He recently began to go barefoot in his room and then into other areas of the home. It is now a daily struggle to get him into shoes and socks. The staff has warned him that he will not be allowed shoeless in the dining room, but he often manages to get to his table without being spotted. Once seated, he is verbally abusive if staff members try to get him back to his room and into shoes.

Apart from the impropriety of a barefoot resident wandering through the home, the nursing staff is afraid that Mr. Rand will sustain some cut or bruise that will develop into a major medical problem. His diabetic condition is quite serious, and he has already had a number of troublesome infections. To complicate matters further, Mr. Rand has decided to stop wearing his hearing aid. His resulting high-decibel speech disturbs other residents, who generally shun him. Staff members find the simplest communication with him onerous. Increasingly isolated, he has become angry and aggressive. So far his aggression has been mainly verbal, but he has intimidated one resident sufficiently to have him ask for a transfer to another floor. Staff members are concerned that Mr. Rand will intimidate other residents or that he will eventually become physically aggressive. In an attempt to deal with these problems, the Director of Nursing asks Mr. Rand if he would be willing to talk to a psychiatrist. He flatly refuses. "I don't want anyone running *my* brain," he says.

Is the Autonomy/Beneficence Framework Sufficient?

These two cases suggest some of the ways that independence can conflict with safety in long-term care. In both cases, care providers might adopt a waiting strategy, but neither safety nor independence will be well served if protective services must step in and rescue a badly incapacitated Mrs. Marner from her apartment or if Mr. Rand's care providers find themselves treating a resident he has assaulted or a nonhealing foot wound he has dealt himself. On the other hand, Mrs. Marner does not want to leave her apartment or receive more home care assistance, and Mr. Rand is equally adamant about going his own rough way.

In standard bioethical discourse these two cases present "classic" conflicts between autonomy and beneficence. The guiding bioethical consensus about such conflicts holds that the autonomous and informed choices of competent individuals should be respected, even if others consider these choices risky or unwise. Care providers' concern for the well-being of patients ought not become coercive or controlling. Patients should remain free to choose against good advice—indeed to define the very meaning of "good" in personal and idiosyncratic terms, even when this cuts against the common wisdom of family members, individual care providers, or the health care system at large.

But while this ethical analysis keeps providers from forcing treatment on unwilling patients, it offers limited guidance in long-term care where decisions about medical treatment make up only part of autonomy's complex terrain and where a "noninterventionist" approach overlooks the supportive and enhancing tasks of chronic care (*Gerontologist*, 1988; Hofland, 1990). In essence, the autonomy/beneficence framework of acute care imposes a decision-making model that is both conceptually and pragmatically narrow, better suited to patients making decisions about specific medical treatments than for residents or clients shaping the ongoing course of their lives in nursing homes and community settings (Agich, 1990, 1993, Chap. 6; Arras, Chap. 10). The acute care model of an isolated agent rationally weighing treatment outcomes does not capture such things as the nature of family involvement, the dynamic, open-ended, vaguely defined, often subsurface choices that characterize long-term care, the ongoing opportunities for the elderly and their care providers to negotiate partial solutions, to *inch* their way along into agreement and understanding (Horowitz, Silverstone, and Reinhardt, 1991; Moody, 1992; Lidz, Fischer, and Arnold, 1992).

Finally, the terminology of choice in long-term care, "independence" and "safety," deserves conceptual inspection in its own right rather than quick translation into the standard autonomy/beneficence framework. Such translation grants conceptual hegemony to acute care, suggesting that independence and safety are polar values and that care providers must invariably choose between them. In contrast with this view, I will attempt to show that safety and independence reveal some deep family resemblances, commonalities that can challenge narrow definitions and forced moral choices.

Safety: Calculating Its Moral Force

In the broad sweep of human history, safety has hardly been a notion to stir speculative theory or stoke revolutions. "To live *safely*" is something of a minimalist's dream, a pale and cautious aspiration when compared with the desire to live freely, or deeply, or passionately. On the other hand, the world is unpredictable and devouring enough to make safety a compelling human goal under certain conditions. In a room suddenly filling with smoke and cries of fire, we are not likely to ruminate on how philosophically narrow a value safety is.

This would suggest two lines of reflection for long-term care. First, safety ought to be understood within the context of other values. In itself, it provides an extremely limited ethical framework. Secondly, an ethically accurate view of safety would require that we look beyond generalities to particular instances. We have to know the *particular* measure of a harm to know the advantage of being safe from it—or the obligation to protect others from it. In practice, then, safety offers little generalized ethical guidance. It is not a value that automatically overrules the risky choices or behavior of the elderly. Risks have to be weighed in terms of concrete benefits and harms. As a goal of care, safety has to be tested against other goals; care providers' estimates of risk have to be measured against the elderly's own estimates; *potential* harms have to be gauged by solid predictors, not worst case scenarios.

In short, safety is not some absolute, always preemptive mandate. It is one value among many, a value whose force shifts and modulates with circumstances, with the goals and motivations of individuals, with their willingness to bear specific burdens, to take on and struggle against specific threats.

Medical versus Psychosocial Definitions

When it comes to deabsolutizing safety in this fashion, the medicalization of long-term care (Estes and Binney, 1989) is a large obstacle. Just as the medical model neglects the social factors in dementia for a tight focus on somatic pathology (Lyman, 1989), so too it fixes on the somatic aspects of safety, overlooking the psychosocial aspects. As a result, some ethically significant questions go unasked: Do concerns for safety and concerns for independence have a common source? Does protecting the elderly from physical harm have a counterpart in protecting them from psychosocial harm? Should harms to mind and spirit count as heavily as bodily harms? Should care providers recognize that safety reaches beyond physical safety?

In Mrs. Marner's case, for example, a psychosocial definition of safety would suggest that her cats, the boxes of her dead sister's belongings, the dirty, poorly equipped, but familiar apartment, even the parasitic companionship of Charley, may be haven and safe harbor to her. And "safe harbor" is no mere figure of speech here. It presses us to think about safety in terms of broad quality-of-life issues, in terms of those things that sustain Mrs. Marner's sense of security, her continuity with the past, and her ability to keep her life from unraveling in the face of frailty. As Agich (Chap. 6) suggested, autonomy should not be viewed simply within the paradigm of clearly defined medical risks and conflicts. In Mrs. Marner's case, the danger of a fall at home has to be weighed against the risks of institutionalization: fractured patterns of living, emotional pain, and social disability. Her physical safety has to be understood in a continuum with other "safeties": the security of familiar routines and places, the mix of order and spontaneity that is her own daily doing, the self-definition and self-esteem that come from enduring roles and relationships, from a sense that she still lives in touch with her past.

These "psychological safeties" do not support the standard polarity between independence and safety. On the contrary, they suggest a basic intertwining in which independence is a primal form of safety, a way to make the world safe for the self, to secure ourselves against the fragmentation, the assorted tyrannies that circumstances, or human systems, or other individuals, even well-intentioned caregivers, might introduce into our lives. Thus, safety is not a matter of physical protection alone. It touches on issues far more foundational to biomedical ethics and especially critical to the development of long-term care ethics.

Safety and Suffering

The chief foundational issue I have in mind here is the issue of suffering, particularly as it has been approached by Eric Cassell (1991a, 1991b). Cassell sees the primary goal of medicine to be the relief of human suffering. And for him this is not some noble sentiment, a high ideal *presumably* beating at the heart of medical practice. On the contrary, he sees relief of suffering as a problematic mandate, a curt reminder that medicine's intense focus on "hard" clinical data often leaves it insensitive to the inner, personal experience of illness and disability. In Cassell's critique, the theme of *patient as person,* that essential configuration voiced two decades ago by Paul Ramsey (1970), still has an indicting edge.

While admitting the success of clinical medicine, Cassell faults it for disregarding suffering—an experience rooted in perceived threats to personal integrity. Suffering arises when the intactness, the inner logic or "hold" of our lives begins to come apart, when we sense we are losing the struggle to prolong into the future the order of our past lives, the integrity of our past selves. For Cassell, suffering is an elusive datum. It does not provide the kind of clinical evidence found in the physical symptoms of disease and illness. To respond to suffering, then, physicians must develop new modes of diagnosis. They must learn to read patients' struggle with the inner disorder and disintegration that illness brings.

Transposed to long-term care and the discussion of safety and independence, Cassell's approach to suffering would require us to look beyond the so-called "hard" data (the risk of injury or some other medical complication) to the "softer" personal data (the struggle of individuals to protect themselves from psychological and moral threat). From such a perspective, "noncompliance" shows some unusual variation. The elderly who take risks, who reject protective advice and services, for example, may in fact be searching for another form of safety. They may be struggling to keep the security of familiar places and patterns, to protect themselves from dislocation and diminishment, to mark off their own areas of control, just as Agich suggests in his description of *actual* autonomy in the previous chapter.

To the extent that this is so, individuals such as Mrs. Marner and Mr. Rand are pursuing alternate calculations of safety and risk—calculations that count some physical and medical risks of less concern than risks to the inner balance of the self. Such calculations are critical ones in long-term care where patients must come to terms with conditions that cannot be cured, conditions that are not episodic "outside" threats but disabilities lodged permanently within their lives (Jennings, Callahan, and Caplan, 1988). In making their own calculations of safety and risk, patients are trying, then, to fathom the shoals of permanent, often progressive, disability. They are trying to make sense of their suffering. This sense can be elusive, chambered in the patient's self, something that care providers must interpret from clue and indirection. But a willingness to take on such interpretation can give providers a morally expansive context for dealing with issues of safety.

Within this context Mrs. Marner's choices may be seen as attempts to preserve a personal world which she feels is slipping away from her. In a very real sense, then, she *is* concerned about her safety, but in a context where high blood pressure and broken bones are less worrisome than fractures to the self. Realizing this, care providers might be able to voice their own concerns for her physical safety in a way that would be more convincing to her. If this fails, they might at least be able to understand and empathize with her on the path she is charting through her suffering, a path they might regret yet still respect.

The primary question would be, then, not how to keep Mrs. Marner safe in a physical sense, but how to help her deal with the whole range of threats gathering around her. To respond to her in this way, care providers would have to develop what Cassell (1991b) calls an "aesthetic" reading of her suffering. They would have to understand the personal order and harmony she has constructed in her past life and the dissonance she struggles with now. No focus on safety narrowly conceived will accomplish this; only a deeper kind of interpretation, a "thick description" of the safety she wants, a sense of the "larger opus" of her life will do here (Aumann and Cole, 1991; Lynn, 1991).

"Mere Independence" versus a Wider Definition

If safety is often a narrowly defined, morally thin notion, so too is independence, especially when it is paired off against safety. In its thinnest form, independence can mean little more than staying out of a nursing home. Independence is thus defined by site, and not by the wide range of quality-of-life considerations important to the elderly themselves. So defined, independence is consistent with frail elderly living in isolation, with few formal services, dependent on informal caregivers whose skills, resources—even willingness to help—may be meager. At this point independence has become "*mere* independence": avoiding the nursing home but struggling on in the community with lean possibilities and limited options (Cohen, 1988).

When independence is so meagerly defined, community-based care is left with impoverished notions of autonomy and diminished quality-of-life goals for its clients. Such a definition also suggests that independence is lost in a nursing home, that if it survives at all, it does so "problematically," as an incubator for noncompliance. In this view, independence means "standing alone" or "standing against," cutting oneself off from others or working against their concerns for one's well-being.

But independence need not be construed in such a self-isolating and confrontational fashion. When we become old and frail, we may still want to go our own way, but that will not necessarily mean we are speaking some elemental "no" to care providers and their concerns. Even if our independence brings us to the thin edges of safety, it may be because we want to live in our own homes with the people (and pets) we have known, with familiar furniture and foods, wearing the clothes we want, washing or not washing as it suits us, and going out or staying put as we please. In an institutional setting our independence will be charted with similar preferences: access to a favorite chair, to the telephone, or to a friend two floors away. We will want the freedom to follow our own inner clocks for eating and sleeping and for getting up and moving about. From our perspective, being independent is likely to mean charting our own way through the minute and mundane realities of daily life (Agich, Chap. 6; Kane and Caplan, 1990, 1993). It will hardly mean some Promethean isolation from others, a declaration of freedom from all the varied ties that inescapably (and supportively) link us to others.

Our perceptions of independence may still, however, not match those of our care providers. A highly medicalized, protectionist, risk-wary model of care may make them focus primarily on the potential harms that independence can bring: injury, poor nutrition, missed medications, disruptive behavior, and poor personal care. And they may well envision the family members and government regulators who will circle fiercely around these harms. From their perspective, our independence may seem a meager counterweight, especially when it seems to be directed at the small-scale stuff of daily life.

Here we confront one of the critical insights in the recent discussion of long-term care ethics. It is precisely in the quotidian choices of life that the elderly secure—or lose—the world as their own. In chronic care, autonomy is more often a matter of negotiating small freedoms than deciding about feeding tubes (Agich, 1993, Chap. 6; McCullough et al., Chap. 11). In dealing with Mr. Rand, for example, the nursing home staff is liable to face continuing standoffs as long as his behavior is interpreted simply as noncompliance. It might be possible, however, to work out some negotiation and accommodation if staff members perceive his behavior as a struggle to maintain the order of his life, to secure himself within this new environment, to mark off his own safe standards in the midst of the institution's enveloping power.

Cutting his own independent path may be the only way Mr. Rand can see himself safe in the nursing home. Realizing this, his care providers might be able to open up some avenues of negotiation with him. They might be able to strike some initial, small-scale pacts about wearing shoes—or a hearing aid. On the other hand, all attempts in this direction might fail. Mr. Rand may prove unreachable, unreasonable, and resistant as stone. Despite their efforts to understand his suffering and struggle, in the end his care providers may still be pressed into a stark choice between his safety and his independence. But then this choice will be informed by these very efforts to gauge his perceptions and motivations. In short, his care providers will have *journeyed* to this final hard choice, not peremptorily begun with it.

Safety, Independence, and Decisional Capacity

The case of Mr. Rand raises one of the most complicating issues in long-term care: the assessment of decisional capacity. If he is indeed unreachable and unreasonable, his care providers face serious questions about his autonomy. Someone who cannot understand or evaluate a risk cannot responsibly bear its burdens. If Mr. Rand's problematic behavior is complicated by cognitive or judgmental deficit, then his care providers bear special responsibility to ensure his safety and the safety of others.

The principle of care providers' responsibility can be difficult to apply in practice, however, because assessing the mental capacity of the elderly is a difficult and obstacle-ridden undertaking. Historically inherited cultural stereotypes, described earlier by Holstein and Cole in Chapter 2, can cloud these assessments, suggesting that the frail elderly are *in general* incapacitated, *by and large* unable to understand, weigh, and take responsibility for risks. Even when these biases have been carefully checked, assessments remain difficult. Elderly in the latter stages of Alzheimer's disease or comparably devastating conditions may have clearly lost all decisional capacity, but for massive numbers of the elderly decisional capacity is often a varied and shifting reality. In these elderly capacity can fluctuate over time. It can be obscured by poor communication or by asocial and eccentric behavior. Most importantly, it can be present in certain areas of choice and behavior but absent in others.

Assessing capacity requires that care providers identify the fluctuations and specific arenas in an individual's capacity, overcome potential communication barriers, and distinguish eccentricity from deep unreasonableness. This can be a long and time-consuming business, and also a technically imprecise one, because it is an attempt to gauge *moral* agency as distinct from cognitive skills or agency, to decide whether an individual can still formulate and follow goals, appreciate risks, and assume the burdens as well as the benefits of independence. Assessing this complex of abilities means more than measuring general intelligence or information-processing skills. It is a matter of gauging individuals' moral agency, in particular their capacity to calculate the darker aspects of their choices and to take responsibility for the harms their behavior might breed.

In this light the task of assessing decisional capacity can be ethically discomforting, disarming even. But discomfort, since it can engender caution, is perhaps a better approach to judging someone else's moral agency than overweening confidence. Moreover, even though there is no technical, ethically "safe" way to judge moral agency, the path of caution is not without purpose or process. In this regard, recent explorations of the "values history" (Caplan, 1992; Doukas and McCullough, 1991; Gibson, 1991) can prove helpful to care providers. The values history provides a format for exploring patients' underlying values and preferences, their sense of reasonable risk, and their own hierarchy of "safeties." As Kane (Chap. 5) and Laurence McCullough and his colleagues (Chap. 11) suggest in this volume, a formal process for inquiring about values gives providers an opportunity to explore with the elderly their own understanding of independence and safety, as well as the priorities which provide the context for their own choices and behavior. In supplying a baseline of information about an individual, a values inventory can aid the process of assessing decisional capacity, particularly by helping providers decide whether a particular risk-laden choice is authentic or unauthentic, reasonable or unreasonable by the individual's own standards.

The Regulatory Framework

Any discussion of the issues of independence and safety in long-term care must take into account the impact of the regulatory system, a system that takes a protective stance toward the elderly and a generally adversarial stance toward their care providers (see Wilson, Chap. 3). In practice, the protection of the elderly produces a much sharper focus on issues of safety than on issues of independence. The recent government regulations on the use of restraints (Collopy, 1992; Evans and Strumpf, 1989) are a good case in point. It can be argued, first of all, that the regulatory system's past emphasis on safety contributed to the practice of using restraints in the first place. The system encouraged a value scheme that elevated safety to a near-absolute value, preferring clear and predictable "outcomes" to the foggier business of balancing concrete instances of safety and independence against each other. Restraints provided an easy-to-use, relatively inexpensive, highly efficient response. Unfortunately, the behavior that restraints "quieted" was often psychologically and socially complex. In effect, the posey vest was a quick technological fix to an intricate ethical problem.

The context for this technological fix was the perceived regulatory mandate that nursing homes should be injury-free, fall-free, disturbance-free environments. Within this context the 1989 Health Care Financing Administration's prohibition on the routine use of restraints struck many care providers as a puzzling turnabout. The regulatory system that had encouraged this practice through its constant stress on safety seemed suddenly to be reversing itself. The puzzlement of providers cannot be attributed solely to some standing opposition to regulations. In the conciseness standard for such mandates, the antirestraint regulations called for change without creating the kind of explicatory context that would provide understanding and motivation (beyond the threat of regulatory sanction, that is). There was no reexamination of safety as a ethical and legal mandate, no clear indication that the system was refining its basic notions of safety and protection, that it might be willing to allow the elderly (and their care providers) to take on certain risks. Because it provided no well-developed moral and conceptual context, the new regulation left many care providers perplexed about how the counterweights of safety and independence were shifting within the regulatory system.

Because of this perplexity, the reform of restraint practice has had a relatively contained impact. It has not fostered much reflection about the basic definitions of safety and independence operative in long-term care. Nor has it sparked much discussion about the effect of regulation on the ethical categories and decision-making processes of providers. Yet these are critical matters for the evolution of long-term care ethics. Unfortunately, the present inspection and review processes are geared to catch poor performance rather than to explore and develop innovations in care practice (Cooney, 1991). In general, the regulatory system shows little interest in engaging care providers in common reflection on ethical problems (e.g., the conflicts that can develop between safety and independence). Care providers, in turn, tend to view regulation as burdensome and adversarial. They see it as a system sharp-eyed for infractions but slow to develop common moral frameworks or programs to educate long-term care staff (Day and Klein, 1987). The net result is a culture of care that is highly risk-aversive.

On the other hand, the "provider industry" is often slow to respond and largely reactive when it comes to ethical issues. Providers have not yet clearly seized the ethics agenda as their own—with the result that the initiative in this area comes largely from regulators and advocates for the elderly. Indeed, when regulators issue broad guidelines, providers are liable to ask for more explicit instructions, as happened when providers recently pressed HCFA to be more specific about the implementation of the Patient Self-Determination Act (Sabatino, 1993). In looking for even more specific instructions, providers were protecting themselves from possible regulatory sanction, but they were also muting their own moral agency, settling for a kind of "cookbook ethics" in which the ethical calculations of care are made by regulators.

Caring for elderly who pursue their own independence, elderly like Mrs. Marner or Mr. Rand, requires that providers develop the kind of ethical reflection that is not easily cookbooked. Kane's caution in Chapter 5 against "cookie cutter" care plans applies forcefully here. But when providers are fearful of triggering regulatory sanctions at every turn, such reflection withers. Micromanagement by the system's rules, or the system's *perceived* rules, takes the place of care providers' moral agency. Ethical reflection cedes to the strategies of risk management or damage control. Mrs. Marner becomes a "safety problem," Mr. Rand a "behavioral problem." In both cases, keeping the resident or client safe also keeps the provider safe.

Such an approach technologizes ethics, turns it into a strategic tacking through regulations rather than a struggle with moral ambiguity and dilemma. There are few signals that this is about to change. The system is still reluctant to grant much moral discretion to providers. It still tends to reduce ethics to "following the regs," still suggests that the vulnerable elderly's surest protection lies in the letter of the law.

Conclusion

But the letter of the law often produces a rigid and minimalist kind of protection. It defines safety and independence in narrow terms, sets them off as "natural enemies," and presses providers to choose between them. A central claim of this chapter, indeed of this volume, is that long-term care is better served by thinking and practice that moves beyond such polarized, bunkered definitions and the either/or decision making they generate.

In dealing with the intricacies of independence and safety it is crucial that long-term care adopt an expansive perspective, one that admits the hazards of life, the risks of autonomy, the moral dilemmas inherent in human frailty—and in human caregiving. In this perspective safety and independence make sense in relation to an individual's *many* values and *particular* goals, in terms of a complex self who may very well autonomously subordinate medical goals and physical protections to other personal ends. Thus, care providers must search for the underlying sources of risky behavior in the elderly, must seek to plumb the noncompliant person's suffering, to find some common ground of understanding. Either/or choices between safety and independence represent positions of last resort. The search for shared understanding, for accommodation, and for tolerable even if not perfect solutions comes first. The underpinning for such an approach is, of course, a kind of conceptual largesse, a perspective that would not position safety and independence as fierce opposites but would see them as values tightly interwoven and mutually illuminating.

REFERENCES

Agich, G.J. (1990). Reassessing autonomy in long-term care. *Hastings Center Report, 20*: 12–17.

Agich, G.J. (1993). *Autonomy and Long-Term Care.* New York: Oxford University Press.

Aumann, G.M.-E., and Cole, T.R. (1991). In whose voice? Composing a lifelong song collaboratively. *Journal of Clinical Ethics, 2*: 45–49.

Caplan, A.L. (1992). Can autonomy be saved. In A.L. Caplan, *If I Were a Rich Man Could I Buy a Pancreas?* pp. 256–281. Bloomington, Ind.: Indiana University Press.

Cassell, E.J. (1991a). *The Nature of Suffering.* New York: Oxford University Press.

Cassell, E.J. (1991b). Recognizing suffering. *Hastings Center Report, 21*: 24–31.

Cohen, E.S. (1988). The elderly mystique: Constraints on the autonomy of the elderly with disabilities. *Gerontologist, 28*(Supplement): 24–31.

Collopy, B.J. (1992). The use of restraints in long-term care: The ethical issues. Washington, D.C.: American Association of Homes for the Aging.

Cooney, L.M. (1991). More professionalism, less regulation. In M.S. Donaldson, Harris-Wehling, J., and Lohr, K. (eds.), *Medicare: New Directions in Quality Assurance*, pp. 18–21. Washington, D.C.: National Academy Press.

Day, P., and Klein, R. (1987). The regulation of nursing homes: A comparative perspective. *Milbank Quarterly, 65*: 303–347.

Doukas, D.J., and McCullough, L.B. (1991). The values history: The evaluation of the patient's values and advance directives. *Journal of Family Practice, 32*: 145–153.

Estes, C.L., and Binney, E.A. (1989). The biomedicalization of aging: Dangers and dilemmas. *Gerontologist, 29*: 587–596.

Evans, L.K., and Strumpf, N.E. (1989). Tying down the elderly: A review of the literature on physical restraint. *Journal of the American Geriatrics Society, 37*: 65–74.

Gerontologist. (1988). Autonomy and Long Term Care. *28*(Supplement): 1–96.

Gibson, J.M. (1991). National values history project. *Generations, 14*(Supplement): 51–64.

Hofland, B.F. (ed.). (1990). Autonomy and long-term care practice. *Generations, 14*(Supplement).

Horowitz, A., Silverstone, B.M., and Reinhardt, J. P. (1991). A conceptual and empirical exploration of personal autonomy issues within family caregiving relationships. *Gerontologist, 31:* 23–31.

Jennings, B., Callahan, D., and Caplan, A.L. (1988). Ethical challenges of chronic illness. *Hastings Center Report, 19*(Special Supplement): 1–16.

Kane, R.A., and Caplan, A.L. (eds.). (1990). *Everyday Ethics: Resolving Dilemmas in Nursing Home Life.* New York: Springer Publishing Co.

Kane, R.A., and Caplan, A.L. (eds.). (1993). *Ethical Conflicts in the Management of Home Care: The Case Manager's Dilemma.* New York: Springer Publishing Co.

Lidz, C.W., Fischer, L., and Arnold, R.M. (1992). *The Erosion of Autonomy in Long-Term Care.* New York: Oxford University Press.

Lyman, K.A. (1989). Bringing the social back in: A critique of the biomedicalization of dementia. *Gerontologist, 28:* 597–605.

Lynn, J. (1991). Commentary on "In whose voice?" *The Journal of Clinical Ethics, 2:* 49.

Moody, H.R. (1992). From informed consent to negotiated consent. In *Ethics in an Aging Society,* pp. 158–183. Baltimore: Johns Hopkins University Press.

Ramsey, P. (1970). *The Patient as Person: Explorations in Medical Ethics.* New Haven, Conn.: Yale University Press.

Sabatino, C.P. (1993). Surely the wizard will help us, Toto? Implementing the Patient Self-Determination Act. *Hastings Center Report, 23:* 12–16.

IV RETHINKING FAMILY ROLES AND RESPONSIBILITIES

CHAPTER EIGHT

What Do Husbands and Wives Owe Each Other in Old Age?

Nancy S. Jecker

What are the ethical responsibilities of a spouse whose partner suffers from a chronic disabling disease? For example, may a loving wife or husband relinquish caregiving responsibilities for a partner who has been disabled by a stroke and is no longer able to speak, move, or swallow? If so, on what basis does one distinguish between meeting and abandoning responsibility? When does shouldering monumental caregiving tasks become self-destructive or self-effacing rather than laudatory? And how do different disease conditions modify the answer? Does it make a difference if a loved one suffers mental, rather than physical, impairments? For example, is it harder or easier to justify placing in a nursing home a partner with an irreversible and progressive dementia, such as Alzheimer's, who no longer understands his or her situation or recognizes family members? What do marriage vows mean anyway, and under what circumstances can persons ethically alter or revoke them? These ethical questions concerning caregiving arise, in part, because of a long history of spousal caregiving in the United States (Holstein and Cole, Chap. 2), reinforced by government policies (Wilson, Chap. 3).

This chapter addresses the ethical nature and limits of the formal, legally recognized marriage between a man and a woman by focusing on relationships among elderly spouses who have been married for a considerable part of their adult lives. Although some of what I claim bears relevance to younger married partners and to newly married elderly spouses, I will not develop or discuss this at any length. Nor will I elaborate the implications that the discussion has for nonmarried partners in long-term heterosexual or homosexual relationships. Throughout my concern is with what is owed to the average husband or wife in an intact and reasonably good relationship. I will not consider what, if anything, is owed when serious offenses, such as physical or psychological abuse, have been committed. All of these topics merit more attention than they have so far received and constitute part of a larger discussion of familial ethics in long-term care decision making. A more complete discussion would encompass not only spousal relationships, but also sibling relationships, parent-child relationships, and various nontraditional relationships.

Why We Need an Ethical Analysis of Marriage

At first we want to be romantic; later, to be bearable; finally, to be understandable. (Bogan, 1992, p. 71)

Questions about ethical responsibilities in marriage challenge us to turn a critical eye on our most intimate relationships with other persons. Examining intensely personal relationships in this way is something we are apt to resist. We may find mystification of love relationships romantic, or fear that rational dissection and analysis will be their undoing. Alternatively, loving relationships might be assumed to defy rational scrutiny altogether. Or it might be thought that the strong feelings of love and connection that underlie intimate relationships are enough to carry people through tumultuous times, making ethical forethought unnecessary.

Despite an inclination to resist applying ethical analysis to marital relationships, our tendency to hold these relationships immune from ethical reflection is ill-advised. Doing so poorly prepares us to face the inevitable hard choices these relationships pose. Far from "coming naturally," our response to wrenching and complex problems in marital life will often require our deepest moral reflection and discipline. In loving relationships, unlike relationships with acquaintances or strangers, we feel the constant tug of strong emotions. We perceive, without exaggeration, that our choices are momentous and will serve as lessons to be passed on to our children. How well or poorly we handle marriage can shape the fate of our families and all of our personal life. The partnership at stake may not endure, but it is truly unique and irreplaceable. While these considerations clearly make ethical deliberation more challenging and difficult, they also make it more urgent and important.

This said, it is hard to understand, much less support, the general neglect of ethics in marriage by contemporary moral philosophy. What attention has been devoted to family ethics has tended to focus primarily on filial relationships between parents and offspring, while saying comparatively little about the relationship between spouses. The discussion of marital ethics that has occurred places an undue emphasis on sexual ethics and is often preoccupied with topics such as premarital sex and adultery. Little has been written about the ethical responsibilities of marriage partners in old age or about the nonsexual duties marriage partners undertake.

Before turning to discuss ethics in marriage directly, it is important to underscore at the outset that my discussion will make certain limiting assumptions. Ethics in marriage, as I will be using this phrase, refers to ethical considerations relevant to formal, legally recognized marriages as they exist in contemporary Western society. It is hard to set forth a set of necessary and sufficient conditions for this conception of marriage, and I will not attempt this. Instead, I want to indicate briefly a family of features commonly associated with getting married in our society. These include (a) a formal ceremony in which mutual obligations are undertaken; (b) the involvement of two and only two persons; (c) a willingness on the part of the persons involved to have sexual relations with each other and no one else; (d) feelings of mutual love and affection between persons; and (e) legal recognition of marital status and assignment of legal rights and duties (Wasserstrom, 1979). Needless to say, we can readily imagine marriages that lack one or more of these features. Thus, common-law marriages exist without a formal ceremony; marriages take place between persons who lack the capacity or will to engage in sexual relations; and people sometimes marry for reasons of convenience or state without loving each other. For purposes of clarity and simplicity, however, I will assume that the five features listed above are present when I refer to ethics in marriage. I in no way intend to suggest that other forms of marriage are less valid or important.

Ethical Foundations of Marriage

Diverse ethical foundations might be pointed to as forming the basis for ethical responsibilities in marriage.

Commitment to a Relationship

Unlike many other family relationships that arise without the consent of the parties involved, a spousal relationship comes about as a result of each person's voluntary decision. By contrast, children cannot choose whether or not they will have a parent-child relationship or (ordinarily) who their parents will be. Thus, duties of children to parents may spring from sources such as gratitude or love, as Sarah Brakman argues in the next chapter (see also Jecker, 1989), whereas spousal duties may relate to the voluntary decision and commitment that initiates the relationship.

Perhaps the most obvious basis for spousal duties is the promise undertaken during the marriage ceremony. Although marital vows do not make explicit mention of caregiving responsibilities, couples generally do agree to a relationship "for better, for worse, for richer, for poorer, in sickness and in health, till death do us part." Modern variants of the marriage ceremony often retain this promise. Taken quite literally, such a promise creates reasonable expectations that the other person will "be there" in the twilight of life, whatever changes time has wrought. When this promise is counted upon, it gives rise to reasonable expectations: people structure their life around another person and expect that person to be with them in the future.

The consequences of breaking this promise may be more hurtful and disappointing than is ordinarily the case, because the reliance and expectations that such a promise creates are more wide-reaching and profound. Marriage involves a serious promise, a promise whose breech by one party is likely to lead to the infliction of substantial pain upon the other. As Aristotle notes, special bonds of attachment generally heighten expectations and create peculiar vulnerabilities, and "it is a more terrible thing to defraud a comrade than a fellow-citizen, more terrible not to help a brother than a stranger" (Aristotle, 1941, p. 1068).

Still how many married persons imagine, or can imagine, upon entering into marriage the full implications of the vows they utter? How many entertain a vivid picture of their partners' fortunes or health souring? How many consider the possibility of a loved one being robbed of memory or losing the ability to function independently? Do married people in fact expect that their partners will be there no matter what the future brings?

Admittedly, with a strict interpretation, a marital promise means literally what it says: there are no limits or qualifying exceptions. Yet a reasonable understanding of marriage does indeed place limits and permit exceptions. For example, married people are not expected to fulfill duties that they are physically or psychologically not able to meet, remain in relationships that become violent or abusive, or show abiding loyalty to persons who are committed to wicked or immoral ends (Thomas, 1989). Certain circumstances can ethically, as well as legally, justify divorce.

These points suggest that the ethical nature of marriage is defined less by the literal vows couples make than by the underlying commitment these vows convey. Thus, we should not look to the actual words spoken in the marriage ceremony to discern the ethical basis of marriage. Instead, we should search for the broader meaning and significance that the vows represent.

In one view marrying conveys a commitment to support and nurture a certain kind of valued relationship. Although the impetus for making such a commitment may be romantic love, the commitment outlasts romantic feelings. A commitment, after all, represents "more than a fair-weather agreement. Otherwise there is nothing in it that may be tested; there is in fact no real element of commitment" (Graham, 1989, p. 210). Moreover, unlike commitments to other kinds of relationships, a marriage commitment is a commitment to a personal relationship. When one stands in a personal relationship, one holds a particular individual's good as one's own. By contrast, in quasipersonal or impersonal relationships, one's concern is with having a certain kind of relationship or with gaining some outside end (Hardwig, 1989). In the latter instances, the particular person with whom one stands in a relationship is incidental to one's desire.

According to a slightly different reading, marrying does not express a commitment to continue a personal relationship with someone; rather, it produces or brings into existence a committed, personal relationship over time (Graham, 1989). Marrying accomplishes this by creating conditions, social and legal sanctions for example, that make it more likely that people will realize their aspiration to have a lifelong love. Through marrying, people explicitly affirm such a relationship as a shared desire, and affirm an intention to work together to make this desire come true.

Yet what, more precisely, does having a personal relationship mean? How does one know when such a relationship is accomplished? Although in some respects personal relationships resemble impersonal and quasipersonal relationships, they also exhibit distinct features. First, the rules governing impersonal and quasipersonal relationships are more or less explicit and the requirements incumbent upon parties more or less apparent. Thus, a teacher relating to students will be expected to follow certain practices, such as lecturing, holding office hours, and grading assignments. Although every class of students is unique, the general patterns and standards of conduct are fairly clear and repeated with each new group. By contrast, personal relationships unfold in profoundly unpredictable ways. We surprise people we love with important revelations about ourselves and by showing whole sides of our personality that are not publicly known. Even the daily dance of the relationship is more apt to contain spontaneous and unpredictable elements. We laugh and cry with those we love, we engage in horseplay, and we respond with anger. These behaviors and our response to them do not follow fixed rules or patterns. Rather, in personal relationships we may find ourselves swimming in waters where we have never been, charting a course through seas that are both unfamiliar and murky.

A second distinguishing feature of personal relationships is that such relationships involve a series of intimate exchanges. For example, friends share projects, go to some length to help each other, reveal secrets, and engage in troubles talk. By contrast, acquaintances wave when they see each other, discuss the weather, or share what they did over the holiday. Finally, sustaining a personal relationship requires, by definition, continuing to care about and be invested in the good of a specific other. Although persons in impersonal or quasipersonal relationships may resolve to stand by particular persons, they do not necessarily resolve to love or feel regard for them.

How can an individual committed to a personal relationship reconcile that commitment with a serious and disabling illness befalling the other person? Is it ever the case that illness makes fulfilling one's commitment an improbable or even impossible feat? In other words, are there instances where, although it is possible to continue a relationship, it is not even conceivable that one could continue to carry on a personal relationship? Take, for example, a situation in which a wife is unable to control her bodily functions; experiences severe tremors, muscular rigidity, and hypokinesia; and is unable to speak. Here, a husband could conceivably continue loving his wife in a deep and personal way and, despite obstacles, could continue to engage in intimate and spontaneous exchanges with her. Still, doing so may mean forging an entirely new repertoire of intimacies. Physical intimacies will no longer include reciprocal sexual relations but may include hand-holding, feeding, and bathing. Verbal exchanges will not continue to involve the same give and take but may involve reading a story. Spontaneity may remain but be expressed through laughter, grimaces, smiles, or winks.

But what if the qualities that form a relationship that is personal are not mutual and are not reciprocated in any meaningful way? For example, what if a disabled husband no longer recognizes his caregiver as his wife? The disabled spouse may then feel to the caregiver like "a presence, but no longer a companion . . . as though his body has been taken over by some alien being, as in some Hollywood Grade B movie" (Meyer, January 9, 1982). Taking this point further, what if a disabled husband treats his wife as if she were a different person on each new occasion she tends to him? One caregiver who found herself in such a situation expresses its ludicrousness and chaos:

> I have been as many as seven people at one time to him. According to my function and the room I was in, he had me separated into all these different people. . . . He would warn me against the woman who had just given him a bath: "She's a bitch. Watch out for her. Watch out for the old lady who's out in the hall. She's always watching." He would warn me against me—the person he would perceive. He would warn me sometimes if I would kiss him. "Watch out! My wife may find out." (Meyer, January 9, 1982)

Is it possible to love a person who does not know you? Even infants soon learn to recognize their parents and smile and coo at their presence. Even pet cats rub against their owners and saunter over to greet them when they arrive home. How can the commitment to carry out a personal relationship proceed when the possibility of its mutuality is so wholly ruined? Should the caregiver in the above example struggle to carry out seven different intimate relationships? Should she attempt to be the seven different people her spouse perceives? If she does, can we call the fractured relationship "personal"? Can we recognize the exchanges as "intimate"?

Clearly there are some kinds of others with whom a personal relationship is not possible. For example, it is not possible to have a personal relationship with inanimate objects, such as works of art; or with places, such as Denver; or with living unconscious things, such as a tree or flower. Certainly it is possible to love such things and to care for and nurture them. It is also possible to respond spontaneously to them, with joy or aesthetic feeling, for example. But the dance of relationship in which we partake remains a solo performance, and no response is ever elicited in the object. In the case of severe dementia, a dance of two may endure, but are the exchanges that are carried out intimate? Consider the following example.

CASE I

Rae had battled carcinoma of the breast for a decade and now had an inoperable bowel obstruction. Discharged from the hospital, she had been told by the medical team "There is nothing more we can do for you." She went home to a hospital bed and bedside commode placed in the living room and waited for death, wished for it to come. She waited for two months, while her spouse of thirty years, Sander, cared for her. She had massive generalized edema and persistent nausea; her skin broke under the pressure of fluid and had to be taped in places. She began a course of morphine a week before the Thanksgiving holiday. That was when she first began to experience episodes of delirium. Rae saw spiders on the walls, hurled objects across the living room, spoke of imaginary persons. These episodes became more frequent until finally, in the end, she ceased to recognize Sander altogether.

In reflecting on this case, one wants to say that the personal relationship between Sander and Rae had ended before the event of Rae's death. Its ending was a process beginning with Rae's delirium and becoming final when Rae ceased to have lucid moments. By this point, although Sander tended to Rae with love and attention, the interactions he had with his wife were no longer mutual or close, the relating no longer constituting a shared intimacy.

If this analysis is correct, then the view that sees marriage as a commitment to a certain kind of valued relationship cannot support a duty to care for disabled spouses under all situations. When the valued relationship that one is committed to having with a spouse becomes impossible to fulfill, the commitment is no longer in force. Sander continued to care for his wife, but he was not obligated to do so according to this view. Instead, his conduct was morally praiseworthy; it revealed his courage in the face of loss and his devotion to the memory of Rae.

Love or Friendship

A different source of ethical responsibility in marriage is the present friendship and love that a marriage manifests. This position denies outright that there are marital obligations as such, not grounded in ongoing bonds of affection. It suggests as well that long-married partners can conceivably make much greater demands and have far higher expectations of each other than younger and newly married partners can. After all, even if people can "fall" instantly in love or can be besieged by strong feelings toward each other, a loving relationship does not begin at once. Rather, such a relationship develops only over time and derives, at least in part, from a series of intimate encounters. These include, for example, making private revelations, sharing time and property, having contact with each other's body, becoming involved in shared projects, and entrusting promises and commitments (Graham and LaFollette, 1989).

With a slightly different interpretation, ongoing affection not only grounds marital ethics but also shapes this ethics in a special way. Ethics grounded in love does not consist of rights and duties; instead, the ethical calling that love supports is best characterized in terms of virtues, such as loyalty, honesty, and trust. This is because "We share ourselves with those with whom we are intimate and are aware that they do the same with us"; it follows that "traditional moral boundaries, which give rigid shape to the self," do not apply and that "talk about rights of others, respect for others, and even welfare of others is to a certain extent irrelevant" (Schoeman, 1980, p. 8). Expressed differently, "the lives of those who are close are not separable, to be close is no longer to have a life entirely your own to live entirely as you choose" (Hardwig, 1990, p. 6). Taking this idea further, marriage might be thought of as a spiritual union, in which two individuals are literally joined, and a new entity is created. Thus, in the traditional Christian conception of marriage, husband and wife become one holy union, and their former, separate selves cease to exist (Graham, 1989). If one agrees that close relationships blur, or even obliterate, the traditional boundaries that exist between persons, then a language of rights and duties is indeed misplaced. For rights are traditionally applied to distinct individuals; duties ordinarily presuppose prior acts of consent by particular persons. Furthermore, the motivation for respecting rights and meeting responsibilities is generally the moral requirement itself, whereas those who love each other should be motivated by the love and affection that exists between them (Blum, 1992; English, 1991).

According to both of the above conceptions, persons who have ceased loving their spouses but remain legally married are no longer ethically called upon to show their partners, for example, sexual fidelity. For it is only the value of "loving someone deeply and completely" that makes sexual fidelity "an ideal worth the sacrifice" (Steinbock, 1992, p. 531). Likewise, the initial promise to stay with someone in sickness and poverty remains in force only so long as the relationship that loyalty preserves continues to be characterized by bonds of affection. Therefore, where love withers the ethical responsibilities of partners wither as well. Sustaining conventional social duties in the absence of love is undesirable, a "trap of self-abnegation and sacrifice" (Poirier and Ayres, 1991, p. 104).

To return to the case described previously, such a conception helps to explain why Sander remained ethically indebted to his wife even after a personal relationship with her had ended. He continued to love his wife, although she did not continue to love or even know him. This kind of love is not mutual, and this kind of relationship is not shared or personal. Nonetheless, Sander related to his wife in a manner that was deep and abiding, and she evoked in him potent feelings, images, and memories. It was his love for her that fortified him and made him feel that he must forge on.

Yet, however appealing this perspective may be, it faces a serious difficulty. It cannot explain why Sander continued to have obligations to Rae even if he no longer loved her. But surely the thirty years between them did not mean nothing. Sander was not free to walk out the door and leave his wife alone and bewildered. Even if he could not muster the courage to continue loving her as she deteriorated physically and mentally, he was not ethically free to jump ship.

Commitment to a Particular Person

These reflections suggest a somewhat different reading of the ethical underpinnings of marriage and the need to return to the idea of commitment with which we began. A final account of the source of ethics in marriage sees marriage as founded on a commitment, but not just a commitment to have a certain sort of valued relationship. Instead marriage is, or is in addition, a commitment to a particular person. Thus, Sander's commitment was not only to have a personal relationship with Rae; it was also a commitment to Rae. This can explain why he remained obligated to her even if a special and intimate relationship was no longer possible, and even if he ceased to love her entirely. Marriage commited him to support his wife's welfare and interests; leaving her when she was dying would have betrayed this commitment.

The Meanings of Caregiving

The preceding discussion reveals that the ethical responsibilities of spouses may spring from distinct sources. On the one hand, the promise we make to those we wed may express our commitment to continue a certain sort of loving relationship with them, or our shared desire to bring such a relationship into existence. Alternatively, the ongoing love that marriage relationships exhibit may form the basis for moral assessment based on duties or virtues. Finally, ethics in marriage may be underlain by the commitment each side makes to support the welfare and interests of the other. Yet even if marriage is ethically rooted in love or commitment, how do spouses make caregiving meaningful? How do the ethical sources that help to sustain marriage also shape its meaning in the caregiving context?

In the later stages of dementia, spouses who love and care for demented partners may find that their partners cease to recognize them, lose touch with their past selves and identities, and no longer understand their current situation. This process of deterioration is surely bewildering, terrifying, and degrading to the demented person, yet its end-point has been described as ultimately "merciful" (Smith, 1992). Once demented persons forget their personal history and lose touch with their present predicament, none of their prior self remains to know or grieve this loss.

The situation is quite different for the demented person's husband or wife. When demented persons are no longer able to appreciate their plight, their spouses remain painfully aware that "this is no longer the same person." The substantial loss of personal identity that accompanies severe dementia lends itself to the thought that marital duties at this stage are duties to a past person who no longer exists. Perhaps they become similar to the duties persons have to those who are literally deceased, such as a duty to execute a will faithfully or keep a deathbed promise. In support of this suggestion, some philosophical analyses of personhood hold that persons continue to exist over time only if memory remains intact (Perry, 1975) or only if psychological connections continue (Parfit, 1975). These accounts lend credence to the idea that whatever ethical responsibilities spouses continue to have are to a being that no longer exists.

Yet in reply to this reasoning it can be said that personal identity encompasses not only intrinsic qualities of individuals, such as rationality and memory, but also the relational features individuals possess (Jecker 1990a, 1990b). For example, a partner who no longer retains his memory continues to have the quality of being someone's husband or wife, someone else's father or mother, this person's neighbor, that person's patient. These relational features may not suffice to establish, in a strict and philosophical sense, that the same individual continues to exist over time. Nonetheless they show that an individual's identity in a social sense persists, even survives, despite grave losses. The social sense of personhood underscores the abiding place individuals have in the lives of others.

But how does the ethical relationship between married persons itself change shape when one party loses some of the essential features of his or her former self? Do all previous responsibilities remain in force? Are new ones created? Clearly, the demands of caring for individuals increase in end-stage dementia. Care for such persons "is not just sustenance of the individual's body, but protection of the person. The values, choices, and dignity of the demented are also vulnerable to harm or neglect. The caregiver is the keeper of the psyche as well as the soma" (Martin and Post, 1992, p. 59).

The case described below illustrates that the relationship that remains when one spouse becomes seriously demented may resemble more closely a relationship between parent and child, rather than husband and wife. Reported in the *Washington Post,* this is the story of Helen and Snowden Chambers, a long-married couple in their sixties.

CASE 2

Helen's and Snowden's life together started disintegrating 10 years ago. . . . Snowden . . . worked for the United States Information Agency [and] . . . was a widely traveled, urbane linguist who knew his way around world capitals. Suddenly, on a trip to Europe, he seemed to lose control . . . a man known . . . for his phenomenal memory . . . began writing notes to himself, reminders of his son's or his mother's name. In the following months, his behavior became erratic. He wandered off, became lost, forgot how to get home, suffered blackouts, so that hours later he could not account for his whereabouts or what he had done. . . . [Years later, Helen] learned that [her husband] . . . had Alzheimer's disease. (Meyer, January 8, 1982, p. A1)

[A long and frightening decline had ensued, and at age 68, Snowden] no longer recognized his wife . . . and had [entirely] lost the ability to control his bodily functions. From being the wife of a sick and profoundly disturbed man, Helen . . . became the caretaker of an adult with all the characteristics of a very young child. (Meyer, January 9, 1982, p. A1)

Yet the analogy with the child in this case is not entirely adequate. Although in both parent-child and spousal relationships caregiving involves care and love for a dependent and vulnerable family member, in the case of the spouse the history of the prior relationship informs a different ethical course. The caregiver's concern is not only to care for someone who is child-like and helpless, but also to make sense of the relationship that now exists in light of its history, to find meaning in adversity. How can Helen construe the relationship she now has with her husband in light of what it once was? One view holds that it is the love that endures, and only this that enables the caregiver to carry on with grace and dignity. According to another view it is only the caregiver's reverence for a shared history and relationship, a prior commitment and promise, that summons strength.

The Limits of Caregiving

> Love is not merely a desire to do good to the object beloved . . . it includes, beside the benevolent impulse, a desire of the society of the beloved: and this element may predominate over the former, and even conflict with it, so that the true interests of the beloved may be sacrificed. (Sidgwick, 1981, pp. 244 and 245)

Even if caregiving can be rendered meaningful, this does not yet address the problem of its ethical limits. For example, to what extent can Helen ethically relinquish caregiving for her husband? When can she do less? When must she? Love and relationship can conflict with individuals' interests, sacrificing these to the "society" of marriage. Each of the ethical analyses discussed so far seems compatible with identifying limits to marital responsibility in the event that such a conflict arises. Thus, all are consistent with the idea that marital responsibility ends where responsibilities have become impossible to meet or where competing obligations or virtues take precedence. The accounts premised upon commitment are consistent with the view that commitments can be waived or relinquished by recipients (Post, 1988). The position that holds spouses' ethical obligations to be founded on love and affection permits the possibility that obligations cease when love and affection sour. Yet how, more specifically, do limits to marital responsibility emerge in the context of caregiving? Consider the following additional comments about Snowden and Helen Chambers' case, made by a *Washington Post* reporter covering the story.

CASE 2 (continued)

> Over the last 10 years her life had come to be dominated by her husband and his condition. . . . At 60, Helen . . . says she yearns for the warmth and comfort of a normal human relationship. The times she and her husband looked forward to sharing after their children were grown, the career she had embarked upon, the friendships the Chamberses had cherished—all

shattered by her husband's disease. "My initial reaction," she says, "was what a waste! It is. It's a waste of two people—him and me." Since her husband requires almost constant care, she can leave the house only when she can find someone willing and able to watch and take care of him. One adult son lives in a basement apartment in the house and helps when he can, but he has to be away much of the day. Her other two sons live elsewhere. . . . Theoretically, . . . [Snowden] could be in a nursing home, but . . . [Helen] would have to pay out of pocket between $17,000 and $33,000 annually for such care, an expenditure that would deprive her of any resources to take care of herself in her own old age. (Meyer, January 9, 1982, p. A1)

To avoid these high costs and become eligible for public support through Medicaid, the Chambers would be required to reduce their assets substantially (Omnibus Budget Reconciliation Act of 1993). For example, if they had assets of $150,000 the Chambers would (in most states) have to spend half their assets on Snowden's nursing home costs before Snowden would be eligible to receive Medicaid (Jones, 1993). If the Chambers had devoted money to a son's college education or assisted with a son's mortgage payment, Snowden would not be eligible for Medicaid for three years from the date these assets were dispersed. If monies had been transferred to a trust, the waiting period would be five years. Even supposing Helen and Snowden can overcome these obstacles and receive Medicaid funding, states can later seek recovery from a person's estate for Medicaid expenses. Thus, if the Chambers spent down their assets to receive Medicaid coverage for nursing home care or home and community-based services (or, at the option of the state, any service provided under the state's Medicaid plan), then at Snowden's death the estate left to Helen could be depleted to reimburse the state for these expenses.

Given these financial constraints, Helen's caregiving responsibilities may seem de facto unlimited. Putting her husband in a nursing home may simply not be a financially viable option. Yet neither a promise, nor a commitment, nor ongoing love and affection can support assigning unlimited caregiving responsibilities to Helen. None of these ethical foundations can make moral sense of, much less justify, Helen's and Snowden's predicament.

The Caregiver's Interests

If love and commitment can take us only so far, where should we locate their limits? When can we expect that the ethical foundations of marriage will begin to crumble under the weight of burden that caregiving entails? Even if caregivers' de facto responsibilities are open-ended, when do they ethically exceed what any individual can bear?

Traditional answers to this question in the bioethics literature are for the most part inadequate. Thus, the literature on surrogate decision making for mentally incompetent persons assumes that family members have presumptive decisional authority (Buchanan and Brock, 1989). However, they are advised to act in accordance with what the incompetent individual would have wanted, or if this is not possible, in accordance with the incompetent person's best interests. Thus, taking a partner to a nursing home is justified if this is what the partner would want if he or she became suddenly lucid and able to make a rational decision. Or nursing home care is ethically defensible provided it is in the best interests of the disabled person.

Yet this analysis gives little guidance in situations where a disabled and incompetent patient would have wanted to remain "forever" under his or her spouse's care. And it provides poor direction in instances where it is indeed in the best interests of an incapacitated spouse to remain at home, but home care places undue burdens on caregivers. Studies show that the burden to caregivers is substantial (Zarit, Reever, and Bach-Peterson, 1980), with caregivers experiencing high prevalence rates of depressive symptoms and disorders (Gallagher et al., 1989), triple the normal incidence of self-reported stress symptoms (George and Gwyther, 1986), almost double the normal use of psychotropic agents (Clipp and George, 1990), reduced immune function (Kiecolt-Glasser et al., 1987), and increased susceptibility to health problems (Pruchno et al., 1990). An approach that requires putting the best interests of the disabled spouse first is unwieldy in caregiving situations because it discourages justified self-concern on the part of caregivers. Thus, it elicits guilt whenever caregivers pay legitimate attention to their own needs and interests.

A fuller picture of long-term care decision making would place various options, ranging from occasional respite care, to regular day care, to placement in a nursing home, in the context of the interests of both the disabled person and the caregiver. Reflecting this broader perspective, I have argued elsewhere that family relationships place ethical limits on how far respect for individuals' wishes extends (Jecker, 1991). Rather than picturing the individual as an island, the individual should instead be situated in a family context, and the family's resources should be regarded as a commons, a resource open to all that can be depleted, if abused. Others urge greater recognition of the potential for legitimate conflicts of interests arising within the family (Arras, Chap. 10; Hardwig, 1990; Moody, 1992) and urge health professionals to form effective relationships with caregivers, which enable them to train caregivers in self-care behaviors, provide referrals to health and social agencies, and use appropriate leverage to involve multiple family members in caregiving (American Medical Association, Council on Judicial Affairs, 1993). The theme of limits to caregiving obligations plays a major role in the preventive ethics strategy for long-term care decision making described in Chapter 11 of this book.

As the Chambers' example makes sadly evident, however, many caregivers who find themselves at the end of their physical and emotional stamina lack access to resources and do not perceive viable alternatives to their current situation. Hence, short of spending down assets to become eligible for public assistance, caregivers often feel compelled to continue against their wishes to care for disabled partners. Yet let us imagine for a moment a society and a health care system in which more options were present. How would caregivers then go about making choices and setting ethical limits? Must they go to the brink of their physical and emotional capacity before they are justified in taking their own interests into account? Must they reach this precipice, and risk falling over its edge, before they can ethically say, "No more"?

In response it can be said that although we owe more to those we love, what we owe is circumscribed by our own distinct and separate interests. In this respect, the view that sees close relationships as destroying the boundaries between persons is potentially misguided. Unless it is possible to reconcile this view with the possibility of both parties having distinct and conflicting interests, the tendency will be to recognize only one person's interests as standing for the interests of both. In the caregiving situation, the tendency has been to give precedence to the interests of the cared-for one, while discounting or even ignoring altogether the interests of the caregiver. Likewise, views that premise marital obligations on the commitment married persons make to each other or to a relationship are potentially deficient. Such positions must account for the possibility that the commitments two people make are not always morally sanctioned, even when they are accepted de facto. Thus, "relationships have moral preconditions: certain agreements cannot be legitimately made. They also have moral side constraints: under certain circumstances, even legitimate agreements cannot be met" (Jecker, 1993, p.

89). To the extent that married persons' commitments are a function of unjust or questionable social attitudes and practices, or are at odds with other ethical considerations, the ethical basis of their commitment becomes problematic.

Even a view that regards going to great lengths for those we love to be morally heroic, rather than morally mandatory, requires important qualifications. Although it is occasionally heroic or admirable to subordinate one's own interests in order to go out of one's way to benefit another person, doing so is not always ethically acceptable.

The Caregiver's Projects

So far I have proposed that those who serve as caregivers should not categorically subordinate their own interests to the interests of the cared for. A further constraint might hold that a person's commitments to others, even those the person loves, should not imply forsaking other goals and projects in life. Caregiving frequently compromises a spouse's health and well being, leading to depression, anxiety, frustration, helplessness, sleeplessness, and lowered morale; it frequently consumes a person's energy, leading to physical and emotional exhaustion (Older Women's League, 1989). Hence, it can readily interfere with the pursuit of other life goals.

The problem that the proposed restriction encounters is that we routinely allow, or even de facto require, individuals to make a career out of caring. Thus, women have historically made a career out of parenting offspring (Holstein and Cole, Chap. 2; Wilson, Chap. 3). If such a career is ethically allowed, even touted, it seems inconsistent to deny devoted spouses a similar opportunity. Although cultural scripts assign caregiving to women, it is also possible for caregiving to be a freely chosen vocation, meaning one that persons select when they have other options from which to choose. Under these circumstances, serving another seems compatible with pursuing, rather than giving up, the important goals and projects one has. Under these conditions, caring need not be destructive of identity; it need not entail that caregivers lose sight of their most important aspirations and plans. If this analysis is correct, then choosing a life of caring is not tantamount to deferring uncritically to others or acting reflexively and uncritically to please. Instead, it may reflect a high degree of love for another human being and a deliberate decision to act in light of that love (Friedman, 1991).

However, it might be argued that the situation of caregiving for a disabled spouse is a special case. Spouses would never prefer the circumstances that make this form of caring necessary, that is, the physical or mental deterioration of one's partner. By contrast, spouses do opt to produce and parent children. Indeed, parenting a child is for many the fulfillment of a central goal in life. By contrast, caregiving for a disabled husband or wife is not a goal people ever envision and hope to realize. Yet even those who are drafted into caregiving by sheer necessity can grow committed to caring. Even those who are free to delegate caring to others can prefer and find fulfillment in providing personal caring. Although the tasks of bathing, feeding, toileting, or turning a helpless and vulnerable oldster may not be aesthetically appealing, they can be emotionally bonding and rewarding. With respect to both child care and elder care, caring can be "an end in itself . . . a state that itself can be fully inhabited. While it may [in the case of parenting] serve as a vessel for reaching a remote shore, it is at the same time and above all a vessel in which one can live even when—especially when—there is no destination in sight or in mind" (Gadow, 1988, pp. 5 and 6). This reflection suggests that the meaning of the marriage relationship can be sustained in the face of certain forms of disability, provided that the original picture of romantic love cherished earlier in life can itself undergo profound transformation.

The Caregiver's Self-Respect

Even if we grant that persons can freely choose to make a career out of caring, under what circumstances does such a choice imperil the caregiver's sense of self-worth? Are there some sacrifices that caregivers cannot make while keeping self-respect and personal dignity intact? Previously, it was argued that treatment decisions for a disabled spouse must take into account the caregiver's interests. Therefore, I want now to suggest that commitments to others, even to those we love, should not extend to the point where they jeopardize self-respect.

To elaborate this proposal it is instructive to consider what, more precisely, self-respect means. Self-respect designates persons with "a sure sense of their own worth" (Rawls, 1971, p. 440). According to the Oxford English Dictionary (1971), self-respect refers to possessing "proper regard for the dignity of one's person." Thus, those who display self-respect neither believe that their place in a moral community is below others, nor judge their rights to be less important than the rights of others, nor belittle the plans and projects they set for themselves (Hill,

1991). Self-respect also designates persons who show self-confidence about their ability, as far as it is within their power, to carry out their plans (Hill, 1991). By contrast, those who lack self-respect may feel perpetually unsure of themselves; they may retreat from their own goals and plans, feeling immobilized by their situation.

Caregiving places caregivers' self-respect at peril because it routinely requires deferring to the needs of others. When the needs and interests of others are not only elevated but allowed to eclipse the caregiver's needs and interests altogether, caring has become exploitive. Yet even when this occurs, caregiving may not yet show damage to the caregiver's self-respect. For caregivers may respond with anger and outrage, believing that their welfare and needs deserve consideration. It is only when caregivers succumb to exploitive situations, coming to regard exploitation as fitting, that caring becomes dangerously destructive of the caregiver's self-respect. In such instances, serving others has become servility, because caregivers construe their rightful place in a moral community as lowly (Hill, 1991).

As self-respect is linked to feelings of self-confidence, caregivers whose self-respect is diminished may come to feel trapped by their situation and may be less able or inclined to pursue viable options. As self-respect is interwoven with feelings of self-esteem and self-worth, when self-respect is undermined caregivers may also be more easily coopted to others' purposes. Thus, they may accede more readily to the wishes of the cared-for in carrying out daily routines, agreeing to give up private meals, or Sundays off, or vacation plans, in order to meet the cared-for's wishes. Or caregivers may acquiesce more readily when family members press for transferring additional responsibilities to them.

In these ways, an initial erosion of self-respect can set in motion an avalanche, which builds gradually but brings ultimate devastation. The end-point of this process may be that caregivers feel spiritually and emotionally crippled and cease believing that their own welfare and interests merit concern. In such situations, devoted caregivers have gone to great lengths on behalf of their spouses and have paid an enormous toll. Although frequently distorted by the language of altruism, self-sacrifice under these conditions becomes a nightmare of self-devastation. Although frequently flaunted as an ideal for women, caring labor under these circumstances brings the destruction of women's identity and character.

The Societal Context of Caregiving

I have already alluded to the point that the burden caregiving imposes may perpetuate injustices within the family by riding roughshod over the caregiver's interests and projects or eroding the caregiver's self-esteem and self-respect. It is important now to underscore this point and also to call attention to the fact that wives and daughters make up by far the largest share of caregivers (Wilson, Chap. 3). When a married older person becomes disabled, a female spouse almost invariably becomes the principal caregiver. This is due, in part, to the discrepancy in life expectancy between men and women and to the fact that men usually marry younger women. When spousal caregivers become too frail or ill to perform as sole caregivers, the most frequently enlisted helper is an adult daughter or daughter-in-law (Brody, 1990). All told, two of every three family caregivers to the elderly are women (Stone, Cafferata, and Sangl, 1987). Men tend to assume the role of primary caregiver only when there is no female to do so, and when they do function as primary caregivers, men generally provide less extensive support services than women do (Horowitz, 1985). Although women are more likely than men to perform as primary caregivers, assisting with feeding, bathing, grooming, toileting, meal preparation, housekeeping, and transportation services, both sexes contribute emotional support, financial aid, and linkage services in roughly the same proportions (Horowitz, 1985).

In light of gender disparities in primary caregiving, some caution that concepts of family obligation or debt "can serve as maleficent ideological warrant for the destruction of daughters [and wives]" (Martin and Post, 1992, p. 63; Rapp, Ross, and Bridenthal, 1979). Others warn that contemporary beliefs about family responsibility perpetuate gender inequity and must therefore be abandoned (Osterbusch et al., 1987). As wives are more likely than husbands to function as caregivers, talk about marital ethics and virtue does indeed sound eerily familiar. It is reminiscent of the traditional patriarchal marriage, in which the male head of household represents the family, and the interests of women (and children) are subordinated to him. Applauding wives who devote themselves wholeheartedly to caregiving for disabled husbands is also hauntingly familiar, echoing stereotypical views about women. Thus, women have been considered "guided by their feelings, and especially their attachment to their husbands and children . . . lacking in both the need and the capacity to participate in public life" (Okin, 1982, pp. 87 and 88). In light of this social and historical backdrop, acknowledging ethical limits to caregiving is imperative. Only when the interests of female caregivers are considered on a par with the interests of cared for persons can society avoid reinforcing destructive family values. Only when the self-respect of caregivers is safeguarded can society avoid perpetuating a spurious ideal for women. Gender disparities in the caregiving burden experienced by spouses show that wives experience a significantly greater burden than husbands do (Fitting et al., 1986; Pruchno and Potashnik, 1989; Pruchno and Resch, 1989), a fact with a long history, as described in Chapter 2. This suggests that women in particular should be encouraged to develop greater awareness of the moral legitimacy and importance of setting limits to caregiving. Family members, case managers, health professionals, and others should not only recognize ethical limits to caregiving but should initiate conversations with caregivers about setting appropriate limits, two themes central to this volume (Arras, Chap. 10; Brakman, Chap. 9; Kane, Chap. 5; McCullough et al., Chap. 11; Wetle, Chap. 4).

In addition to justice concerns arising within the family, caregiving simultaneously poses justice concerns outside the family in the larger context of society. Caring labor, both inside and outside the home, has not been borne equally by different groups in society. Historically, it has been performed by women, minority groups, the poor, the lesser educated, and those with the least power. Caregivers often work long hours while earning no or meager wages. They often find their efforts devalued by society and even by the beneficiaries of their care (Kane, 1990). The situation of spouse caregivers raises special justice concerns, because spouses who care are among the most vulnerable of all caregivers. They comprise the largest number of sole caregivers and are typically older, in poorer health, with lower incomes, and provide more intensive care for longer periods of time (Montgomery and Datwyler, 1992).

Societal justice is also at stake when society makes decisions about investing financially in long-term care and helping to underwrite the costs of nursing homes, home care, and community services. At present, the United States devotes relatively few public resources to caring for chronically disabled persons (Wilson, Chap. 3). In 1991, more than 43 percent of nursing home care expenditures were paid out of pocket by individuals and families (United States Department of Health and Human Services, 1993). Society has chosen instead to invest large amounts in acute-care medicine, largely in the form of intensive, short-term, hospital care that is crisis-driven (Jecker, 1995). Some argue for efforts to maintain, or even increase, "free" labor by family members, because without such labor public expenditures would be much higher than they presently are (Rivlin and Wiener, 1988). It is precisely such an attitude that has led to intolerable conditions for caregivers, exemplified by Helen and Snowden Chambers' situation. Helen had scant assistance with caregiving chores, no economic compensation for her efforts, meager opportunity to participate in an outside social life, and little chance to lead a semblance of a normal life.

Caregiving under these circumstances knows no reprieve. It is intimidating and isolating; it breaks the spirit of the carer and ruins the meaning of relationship between the cared-for and caregiver. Although we like to think of individuals and families as self-reliant, reflection on the burden of caregiving fast explodes this myth. Such reflection reveals that families cannot function well or at all as "a closed circle of reciprocal obligations with no public institutions to support it" (Post, 1988, p. 13). A philosophy of self-help has already been tried and failed: it has led to absent or spotty coverage, ruinous burdens, and physical, emotional, and economic hardships for families (Binney and Estes, 1988; Nickel, 1985).

Although such brief remarks cannot do justice to the larger problem of burden sharing, it is imperative at least to mention societal responsibility in tandem with any discussion of family ethics. For both the meaning and ethical nature of the family show the imprint of societal values and decisions. Unless society acts as a brake on family responsibility and shares caregiving burdens more equitably, the idea of family morality will become a moral travesty. Alas, caregiving can stand for moral excellence only when society prevents caregiving from becoming an unwieldy and self-destructive hardship. Caregiving can fulfill moral duties only when society prevents caregiving from leading to unwise and unbearable demands.

REFERENCES

American Medical Association, Council on Scientific Affairs. (1993). Physicians and family caregivers. *Journal of the American Medical Association, 269*: 1282–1284.

Aristotle. (1941). Nichomachean ethics. In R. McKeon (ed.), *The Basic Works of Aristotle*, pp. 935–1112. New York: Random House.

Binney, E.A., and Estes, C.L. (1988). The retreat of the state and the transfer of responsibility. *International Journal of Health Services, 18:* 83–96.

Blum, L. (1992). Personal relationships. In L.C. Becker and C.B. Becker (eds.), *Encyclopedia of Ethics,* Vol. II, pp. 956–960. New York: Garland Publishing Co.

Bogan, L., quoted in Moody, H.R. (1992). *Ethics in an Aging Society.* Baltimore: Johns Hopkins University Press.

Brody, E.M. (1990). *Women in the Middle.* New York: Springer Publishing Co.

Buchanan, A.E., and Brock, D.W. (1989). *Deciding for Others.* New York: Cambridge University Press.

Clipp, E.C., and George, L.K. (1990). Psychotropic drug use among caregivers of patients with dementia. *Journal of the American Geriatrics Society, 38:* 227–235.

Compact Edition of the Oxford English Dictionary. (1971). New York: Oxford University Press.

English, J. (1991). What do grown children owe their parents? In N.S. Jecker (ed.), *Aging and Ethics,* pp. 147–154. Clifton, N.J.: Humana Press.

Fitting, M., Rabins, P., Lucas M.J., and Eastham, J. (1986). Caregiving for dementia patients: A comparison of husbands and wives. *Gerontologist, 26:* 248–252.

Friedman, M. (1991). The practice of partiality. *Ethics, 101:* 818–835.

Gadow, S. (1988). Covenant without cure: Letting go and holding on in chronic illness. In J. Watson and M.A. Ray (eds.), *The Ethics of Care and the Ethics of Cure: Synthesis in Chronicity,* pp. 5–14. New York: National League of Nursing.

Gallagher, D., Rose, J., Rivera, P., Lovett, S., and Thompson, L.W. (1989). Prevalence of depression in family caregivers. *Gerontologist, 29:* 449–456.

George, L.K., and Gwyther, L.P. (1986). Caregiver well-being. *Gerontologist, 26:* 253–259.

Graham, G. (1989). Commitment and the value of marriage. In G. Graham and H. LaFollette (eds.), *Person to Person,* pp. 199–212. Philadelphia: Temple University Press.

Graham, G., and LaFollette, H. (1989). Honesty and intimacy. In G. Graham and H. LaFollette (eds.), *Person to Person,* pp. 167–181. Philadelphia: Temple University Press.

Hardwig, J. (1989). In search of an ethics of personal relationships. In G. Graham and H. LaFollette (eds.), *Person to Person,* pp. 63–81. Philadelphia: Temple University Press.

Hardwig, J. (1990). What about the family? *Hastings Center Report, 20*: 5–10.

Hill, T.E. (1991). *Autonomy and Self Respect*. Cambridge, Mass.: Harvard University Press.

Horowitz, A. (1985). Sons and daughters as caregivers to older parents: Differences in role performance and consequences. *Gerontologist, 25*: 612–617.

Jecker, N.S. (1989). Are filial duties unfounded? *American Philosophical Quarterly, 26*: 73–80.

Jecker, N.S. (1990a). The moral status of patients who are not strict persons. *Journal of Clinical Ethics, 1*: 35–38.

Jecker, N.S. (1990b). Anencephalic infants and special relationships. *Theoretical Medicine, 11*: 333–342.

Jecker, N.S. (1991). The role of intimate others in medical decision making. In N.S. Jecker (ed.), *Aging and Ethics*, pp. 199–216. Clifton, N.J.: Humana Press.

Jecker, N.S. (1993). Impartiality and special relationships. In D.T. Meyer, K. Kipnis, and C.F. Murphy (eds.), *Kindred Matters: Rethinking the Philosophy of the Family*, pp. 74–89. Ithaca, N.Y.: Cornell University Press.

Jecker, N.S. (in press, 1995). Caring for the disabled elderly: The economics and ethics of financing long term care. In J.W. Walters and D.R. Larson (eds.), *Health Care for the Old: Advancing the Debate*. Champaign: University of Illinois Press.

Jones, K. (August 28, 1993). Putting new strings on long-term care. *New York Times*: 29.

Kane, R.A. (1990). Everyday life in nursing homes: "The way things are." In R.A. Kane and A.L. Caplan (eds.), *Everyday Ethics: Resolving Dilemmas in Nursing Home Life*, pp. 3–20. New York: Springer Publishing Co.

Kiecolt-Glasser, J., Glaser, R., Shuttleworth, E., Dyer, C., Ogrocki, P., and Speicher, C. (1987). Chronic stress and immunity in family caregivers of Alzheimer's disease victims. *Psychosomatic Medicine, 49*: 523–535.

Martin, R.J., and Post, S. (1992). Human dignity, dementia and the moral basis of caregiving. In R.H. Binstock, S.G. Post, and P.J. Whitehouse (eds.), *Dementia and Aging*, pp. 55–70. Baltimore: Johns Hopkins University Press.

Meyer, L. (January 8, 1982). Aging prematurely: No cure for illness that strikes elderly. *Washington Post*: A1.

Meyer, L. (January 9, 1982). A family stranger: Irreversible illness alienates victim, afflicts those who care. *Washington Post*: A1.

Montgomery, R.J.V., and Datwyler, M.M. (1992). Women and men in the caregiving role. In L. Glasse and J. Hendricks (eds.), *Gender and Aging*, pp. 59–68. Amityville, N.Y.: Baywood Publishing Co.

Moody, H.R. (1992). *Ethics in an Aging Society*. Baltimore: Johns Hopkins University Press.

Nickel, J.W. (1985). Charity, family aid, and welfare rights. *Logos: Philosophical Issues in Christian Perspective, 6*: 71–77.

Okin, S.M. (1982). Women and the making of the sentimental family. *Philosophy and Public Affairs, 11*: 65–88.

Older Women's League. (1989). *Failing America's Caregivers: A Status Report on Women Who Care*. Washington, D.C.: Older Women's League.

Omnibus Budget Reconciliation Act of 1993. (1993). Public Law 103-66, August 10, 1993. Reported in *Congressional and Administrative News*, Vol. 7. St. Paul, Minn.: West Publishing Co.

Osterbusch, S.E., Keigher, S.M., Miller, B., and Linsk, N.L. (1987). Community care policies and gender justice. *International Journal of Health Services, 17*: 217–232.

Parfit, D. (1975). Personal identity. In J. Perry (ed.), *Personal Identity*, pp. 199–223. Berkeley: University of California Press.

Perry, J. (1975). Personal identity, memory, and the problem of circularity. In J. Perry (ed.), *Personal Identity*, pp. 135–155. Berkeley: University of California Press.

Poirier, S., and Ayres, L. (1991). Stories of family caregiving: Case studies in moral reasoning. *Journal of Medical Humanities, 12*: 97–110.

Post, S. (1988). An ethical perspective on caregiving in the family. *Journal of Medical Humanities and Bioethics, 9*: 6–16.

Pruchno, R.A., Kleban, M.H., Michaels, J.E., and Dempsey, N.P. (1990). Mental and physical health of caregiving spouses. *Journal of Gerontological Psychological Science, 45*: 192–199.

Pruchno, R.A., and Potashnik, S.L. (1989). Caregiving spouses. *Journal of the American Geriatrics Society, 37*: 697–705.

Pruchno, R.A., and Resch, N.L. (1989). Husbands and wives as caregivers. *Gerontologist, 29*: 159–165.

Rapp, R., Ross, E., and Bridenthal, R. (1979). Examining family history. *Feminist Studies, 5*: 174–200.

Rawls, J. (1971). *A Theory of Justice*. Cambridge: Harvard University Press.

Rivlin, A.M., and Wiener, J.M. (1988). *Caring for the Disabled Elderly*. Washington, D.C.: Brookings Institution.

Schoeman, F. (1980). Rights of children, rights of parents, and the moral basis of the family. *Ethics, 91*: 6–19.

Sidgwick, H. (1981). *The Methods of Ethics*, 7th ed. Indianapolis: Hackett Publishing Co.

Smith, D.H. (1992). Seeing and knowing dementia. In R.H. Binstock, S.G. Post, and P.J. Whitehouse (eds.), *Dementia and Aging,* pp. 44–68. Baltimore: Johns Hopkins University Press.

Steinbock, B. (1992). Adultery. In C. Mills (ed.), *Values and Public Policy,* pp. 527–532. Orlando, Fla.: Harcourt, Brace, Jovanovich.

Stone, R., Cafferata, G.L., and Sangl, J. (1987). Caregivers of the frail elderly: A national profile. *Gerontologist, 27:* 616–626.

Thomas, L. (1989). Friends and lovers. In G. Graham and H. LaFollette (eds.), *Person to Person,* pp. 182–198. Philadelphia: Temple University Press.

United States Department of Health and Human Services. (1993). *Health United States 1992.* Hyattsville, Md.: U.S. Department of Health and Human Services, DHHS Publication no. 93-1232.

Wasserstrom, R.A. (1979). Is adultery immoral? In R. Wasserstrom (ed.), *Today's Moral Problems,* 2nd ed., pp. 288–300. New York: Macmillan Publishing Co.

Zarit, S.H., Reever, K.E., and Bach-Peterson, J. (1980). Relatives of the impaired elderly. *Gerontologist, 20:* 649-655.

CHAPTER NINE

Filial Responsibility and Long-Term Care Decision Making

Sarah Vaughan Brakman

It comes as no surprise to practitioners in long-term care settings that children account for a large proportion of caregivers for the chronically debilitated aged (Brody, 1984, p. 736; Older Women's League, 1989, p. 1; Wilson, Chap. 3) and that adult children are often called upon to be the decision makers for the long-term care of parents. Most elderly report continuing contact with at least one of their children (Christiansen, 1987, p. 72). According to the Older Women's League, 31 percent of all women over 18 will care for both children and parents over their lifetime. At least 1.8 million women are simultaneously caring for children while coping with elder care responsibilities, with over half of these women also in the paid labor force. One in five women has a parent living in her home (Older Women's League, 1989, p. 3). Filial responsibility is a crucial aspect of long-term care; yet as Martha Holstein and Thomas Cole observed (Chap. 2), after the early nineteenth century, public discussions on dependency have not emphasized the family's role. Confusion regarding intergenerational expectations, particularly but not solely for women, obtains at the public and family level, causing resentment and anger and raising problems for the planning of care that involves integration of formal and informal supports (Wetle, Chap. 4).

What are the ethical obligations of adult children whose parents are in need of long-term care? Are there certain tasks or specific acts that adult children ought to do for their parents? When is it ethically justified for adult children to end or limit their involvement in "hands-on" caregiving or decision making responsibilities? How can the health care professional help adult children clarify their filial obligations to an elder with long-term care needs?

The conceptual basis of filial obligations is different from that of spousal obligations. As Nancy Jecker (Chap. 8) rightly claims, marital obligations of caregiving are founded on a commitment to a particular person. Parents, however, do not (initially) make commitments to a particular child, but rather to the parent-child relationship. Furthermore, unlike the marriage commitment, there is no meaningful way to say that children have entered *voluntarily* into a *contractual* relationship with their parents. However, both spousal and filial relationships and the obligations that flow from them share a similar feature: persons who are vulnerable to one another in special ways rightly expect that certain of their needs will be met by the other (Goodin, 1985).

In this chapter I present and analyze two leading candidates for the conceptual foundation of filial obligations, reciprocity and gratitude. I argue that such duties are best understood as obligations of gratitude and discuss the implications of the gratitude account for filial obligations of long-term care. The analysis is limited to the traditional, legally recognized parent-child relationship (biological and adoptive), where the parents have provided their children with the basic necessities of life and perhaps have even gone beyond these in some ways to try to raise their children well. While gender differences concerning the amount and more recently the kinds of caregiving provided by female rather than by male children are well known and documented (Older Women's League, 1989, pp. 3 and 4), this analysis focuses on the obligations that any child has to either parent. It does not, as a universal claim of ethics, make distinctions based specifically on gender, and in fact it is a secondary purpose of this analysis to show that overburdening of women is not supported by a conceptual analysis of filial obligations.

Reciprocity and Gratitude

Table 2 shows the most relevant differences between reciprocity and gratitude, and it summarizes the crucial features necessary for both the existence and the fulfillment of obligations on each account.

Reciprocity literally means to return in degree, and often in kind, the benefit that another has bestowed. It is typically characterized by the notion of "repayment" (Becker, 1986, p. 4; Aristotle, 1941). As seen in Table 2, the version of reciprocity that is most likely to be applicable to the parent-child situation may be outlined as an ethical obligation that requires good to be returned for the good received, in degree and possi-

Table 2. Reciprocity and Gratitude Contrasted

Reciprocity	Gratitude
1. Return or repay benefits received.	1. Not repayment
2. Motive of donor not relevant to existence of obligation; may influence degree of return.	2. Motive of donor decisive to existence of obligation: voluntary, intentional, benevolent, and noncoercive.
3. Return in degree and (possibly) in kind of the benefit received.	3. Response ought to be relative to degree of value of benefit as perceived by donor and as determined by motive of donor. When present, the greater the degree of sacrifice by donor, the greater the gratitude obligation.
4. Relationship between the parties may end when obligation fulfilled.	4. Relationship between the parties is furthered by fulfillment of obligation.
5. Attitude of recipient is not relevant for the existence or fulfillment of the obligation.	5. Attitude of recipient is not relevant for *existence* of obligation; attitude is relevant for *fulfillment* of obligation.

bly in kind. Exact or closely proportional repayment is required. The relationship between the individuals may end when the repayment is made, and the motive of the giver is not relevant to whether the duty of reciprocity exists for the receiver. The giver may benefit the receiver either knowingly or unknowingly.

An example of the belief that filial obligations are grounded in a notion of reciprocity is found in Blackstone's *Commentaries on the Laws of England:*

> The duties of children to their parents arise from a principle of natural justice and retribution. For to those who gave us existence we naturally owe subjection and obedience during our minority, and honor and reverence ever after; they who protected the weakness of our infancy are entitled to our protection in the infirmity of their age; they who by sustenance and education have enabled their offspring to prosper ought in return to be supported by that offspring in case they stand in need of assistance. (Blackstone 1856)

Blackstone believed that justice requires reciprocity. Children ought to return to parents the same type of benefits that the parents provided to the children when the parents become similarly in need. But is this really the best way to think about filial responsibility? Consider the following case reported in the *New York Times* (Lewin, 1989):

> Dorothy Shanklin, 52 years old, and Juanita Eubanks, 48 years old, are sisters who care for their 81-year-old mother, Hattie Walker. Hattie is disabled by a stroke. Dorothy and Juanita both work full time and are married. They take turns sleeping in the room with their mother every week, giving her the bed pan, and making sure she doesn't get out of bed unattended and fall. They share the expenses of the attendant who stays with their mother during the day. In addition, Juanita moved into her mother's home with her husband and their 12-year-old daughter. Juanita has said, "I feel good knowing she's getting as good care as a person can get." Both daughters express a sense of pride and love that they can care well for the mother who cared well for them.

In light of this case, filial obligations as a requirement of reciprocity raise at least three troubling considerations. To begin, reciprocity as repayment seems inappropriate for filial obligations. Parents (for the most part) do not give benefits to their children with the expectation of repayment. Indeed, they are often insulted by such thoughts. Parents have been known to say things similar to Hattie Walker, "Lord, isn't it something: my baby's taking care of me just like I took care of her." While Hattie appears to be discussing the "return in kind" from her daughter, she also seems surprised, as if she did not expect it. It is readily imaginable that further conversation with Hattie would reveal that if she found out that her daughters were attempting to "repay" her, she would be hurt and might even reject her daughters' help. What seems important here is that Hattie believes and recognizes that her daughters *want* to help her, but not because they think they *have* to repay her. The notion of repayment does not capture the spirit of the caregiving that Juanita and her sister are providing.

There are those who argue that the mere fact that parents and children do not like to view caregiving duties as repayment, especially when there is a warm and positive personal connection between the children and parents, does not mean that the obligations are not in reality repayment. This implies that it is possible to have an obligation that can never be fulfilled. How could children ever truly "repay" parents? In the case of the reciprocity argument for biological parents, it does not even make sense. What would count as payment for the benefit of having been given life? For caretaking parents who are not also the biological parents of their children, there is the question of what would count as repayment, and, equally puzzling, how would this be determined? How much care should Dorothy and Juanita give to their mother in order to equal what Hattie had done for them? Practically, this answer would be difficult, if not impossible, to obtain. Therefore, it seems unlikely that filial duties would be duties of reciprocity.

Additionally, as seen in Table 2, reciprocity is not sensitive to motivation on the part of the donor or parent. Whether someone provides benefits knowingly or unknowingly or provides benefits in order to secure a relationship, to cement a friendship, to benefit a person, or to make the other person feel indebted does not matter to the existence of the obligation of reciprocity. Filial obligations based on reciprocity are not in any way dependent upon good or positive motivations of parents when they were providing the benefits. This seems troublesome precisely because parental motivation is such an important component of the evaluation of the parent-child relationship. In determining the types or amount of obligations to care that would later fall upon children, it would seem to be important whether parents gave grudgingly to their children or provided them with the best of everything merely so that their children reflected well on them. Such motives, if they were the determining ones, are generally considered to lessen the respect for the individuals who have them. Dorothy and Juanita recognize the voluntary, warm, self-giving that led their mother to take such good care of them when they were little, and this matters to them.

If we turn to a gratitude account of filial obligations, we see that gratitude, like reciprocity, is a response to having benefitted by another's actions. Gratitude, though, is not strictly a repayment for the benefit received. A difficulty presents itself, as it is often said that there is a "debt of gratitude," *as if* it is something that must be repaid to a creditor (Card, 1988, pp. 115–127). Often, when someone does something for another at great personal risk or incurs an unexpected expense or difficulty, even though it was freely done, it is believed that the second person ought to compensate the first for his trouble or his loss (Simmons, 1979, p. 164). It would, however, be considered *un*grateful in such cases, and all others fitting the criteria given for gratitude in the table above, to attempt to repay the giver. This would mean either that one did not recognize the motive of the giver or that her good will is rejected (Berger, 1985, p. 302). Additionally, in most cases in which one has the obligation of gratitude, the concept of making an equal return or repayment for a benefit is inapplicable (Kant, 1797, p. 249). Both of these implications are relevant for filial obligations; many parents, like Hattie, would feel hurt if their children attempted to "repay." If the benefit given by the parents to the child needs to be repaid it may seem that the care, freely given by the parents with the intention to benefit the child, was rejected by the child, and therefore the parents' good will and love were in effect rejected.

Gratitude, better than reciprocity, also seems to capture the relevance of parental motivation to the existence of filial obligations. For gratitude the giver must provide the benefit voluntarily, intentionally, benevolently, and must not force the recipient to accept the benefit. Parents are usually free to provide benefits to children. We assume that, in general, parents have benevolence for their children and that they in general ought to benefit their children primarily for the good of their children.

According to gratitude, the greater the benevolence of the giver the greater is the extent of gratitude; similarly, the greater the value of the benefit, the greater is the extent of the gratitude. The sacrifice made by the giver ought to affect the magnitude of the gratitude response. Again, this feature captures our intuitions concerning the nature of the parent-child relationship. On initial inquiry, it does not seem at all difficult to support the view that the more a parent does that is beneficial for a child, the greater the child's gratitude ought to be. Additionally, while parents make special efforts for their children on a routine basis, if parents sacrifice for their children, the extent of the gratitude response ought to increase proportionally to the degree of the sacrifice made by the parents. Parental sacrifices do not have to be repaid in full or in kind (if that were even possible), but some type of response as recognition appears due.

Another difficulty with basing filial obligations on reciprocity has to do with the status of the morally significant relationship between parent and child. On a reciprocity account, once a duty of reciprocity is met or discharged, the relationship based on reciprocity (debtor to debtee) ends. The status of the original, predebt relationship is restored. The argument that bases all obligations to parents on reciprocity holds that when filial obligations are fulfilled, the morally significant relationship between parents and children terminates. Children will no longer "owe" anything to their parents. What, though, is the status of the parent–adult child relationship before the duty of reciprocity exists? This question is meaningless for solely biological parents because the child, and hence the possibility of any relationship, did not exist prior to the duty. However, even if it were possible to satisfy the demands of repayment, what would the status of the filial relationship be for solely caretaking parents? The status of the relationship before reciprocity was that of strangers.

Can it meaningfully be said that after obligations of reciprocity have been met, children owe parents no more than what strangers owe one another? The answer to this must surely be "no." The emotional and biological bond between parents and children gives the relationship a permanent and central place in children's lives, quite apart from whether a child has succeeded in paying back or returning benefits to her parents (Callahan, 1985, p. 35). It seems absurdly contrived in this circumstance to claim that parents and children could ever again be moral strangers.

With a gratitude account, by contrast, after such duties are met the relationship is not severed but in fact furthered and enhanced. Kant claims that the obligation of gratitude lingers because one will always have cause to be grateful to another for his spontaneous benevolence (Kant, 1797, p. 249). Surely this is true in the case of parents and children. Others have argued that a sincere gratitude response establishes "a relationship of moral community . . . maintained, or recognized, consisting of mutual respect and regard" (Berger, 1985, p. 302). This again captures the complex nature of past dependency and interdependency that characterizes the parent-child relationship.

Not meeting the duties of gratitude may lead away from the formation of such a community or relationship, and it may terminate or prevent a relationship from being formed. This is seen especially when children reject parental benefits because they do not want to be "indebted" and when parents, injured, claim that a child is "ungrateful" when there is a lack of response. The parental injury results from viewing the lack of response as a rejection or indifference to the good will of the parents. At the very least, the fulfillment of obligations of gratitude appears to create, enhance, and reinforce the relationship between the donor and the recipient or between parents and their children. Children and parents are never "free" of their relationship to one another, even if there exists no personal relationship.

A final difficulty with viewing filial obligations as obligations of reciprocity begins with the question of whether reciprocity can be said to be due to those who benefit another when it is in fact their obligation to do so. Why would children have an obligation to repay their parents for the care they received when their parents were merely "doing their job"? Do individuals have an obligation of reciprocity to emergency room doctors who save their lives? The doctors are simply doing their job. Payment is usually made to the hospital, not directly to the doctors. The doctors will get paid whether the ill persons came to the emergency room or not. We do think, perhaps, that the patients may owe the doctors something, but surely not a life-saving or an attempt thereat in return. By the same token, obligations of reciprocity to parents are not owed when it is the job of parents to take care of their children. However, we do in fact think it the duty of parents to take care of their children. This leads to the conclusion, on a reciprocity account, that filial obligations are not present. Since we are assuming that such obligations do exist, this conclusion is not satisfactory.

What, then, does a gratitude account of filial obligations say about this? Gratitude is appropriate in a situation where providing a benefit for the sake of another is the obligation of the person. The claim about the doctors was that something might be due to them. Is not this "something" gratitude? Praise or appreciation may be due the doctors who did their duty because of the effort that was made to do it, the way they carried out their obligation, and/or the great value of the benefit to the doctors and the patients. Gratitude, unlike reciprocity, may be owed even to those who are fulfilling their obligations. The belief that parents have an obligation to take care of their children is not inconsistent with the view that adult children have duties of gratitude to their parents for that care.

These difficulties with reciprocity as the conceptual basis of filial obligations reveal that reciprocity is at best ill-suited to be the conceptual basis of filial obligations. The criticisms show that there are features that are viewed as morally relevant to the nature of the parent-child relationship that are not fully or satisfactorily captured by a reciprocity-based account of filial obligations. However, the gratitude account is capable of capturing these features: filial obligations are at the very least better understood as obligations of gratitude rather than of reciprocity. I now turn to a consideration of what these obligations are and their implications for long-term care decision making.

Filial Responsibility and Implications for Long-Term Care Decision Making

As defined in Table 2, gratitude is the creation of a moral relationship between individuals by the voluntary, intentional, and noncoercive bestowal of a benefit from one to another with a benevolent motivation to aid the recipient. Gratitude itself is a response on the part of the recipient to the generosity of the giver, but what is this response and what does it entail if not repayment? At the very least, a grateful response would be one that demonstrates a positive recognition of the generosity of the giver. Indeed, as we saw earlier, attempted repayment when the above conditions hold effects a rebuff of the giver's intentions. One demonstrates gratitude by performing certain acts in certain ways that show that one values the benefit itself and that one values the giver as the source of the benefit. In fact when we think about gratitude, the acts that are considered to be acts of gratitude admit a transparency to attitudes that motivate them. It is important to Hattie Walker and her daughters that the caregiving is motivated by certain attitudes and not others.

Though there may be others, at least two attitudes readily present as constitutive of the gratitude response. These are the attitudes of appreci- ation and goodwill. Appreciation is a positive attitude possessed by those who have received or perceive they have received something of worth from another. The object of appreciation may be either the benefit received or the benevolence of the giver or the sacrifices the benefactor may have made to provide benefits. In other words, one may be appreciative of receiving a benefit or of the positive feeling that motivated the giver to act.

Goodwill is the positive inclination of the will, including kindly feelings, directed toward another. Unlike appreciation, goodwill can only be directed to another person and not also to the benefit itself. In the case of gratitude, goodwill is the positive attitude that a recipient has toward the benefactor for (a) being the source of a benefit and (b) for the benevolence that the donor has shown. Gratitude for the benevolence or goodwill displayed by a benefactor includes not only appreciation for the benefactor's benevolence but also goodwill directed to the benefactor in return. It is a particular type of goodwill that is secured by the goodwill of the donor. One does not "pay back" the benefit (reciprocity), but rather one responds in kind to the goodwill that the donor has for one. There is, therefore, a reciprocal element of gratitude, but this is not the repayment found in the reciprocity account. One is to have goodwill especially for this other person because he has intentionally benefitted one for one's own sake. In addition to the goodwill one ought to bear others in general, one ought to have a stronger or deeper sense of goodwill for the individual who is also one's donor.

For filial obligations based upon gratitude, this means that adult children ought to cultivate appreciation and goodwill for the benefits that their parents provided and for the parents being the source of these benefits (Weiss, 1985). It is generally believed that one cannot be morally obligated to *feel* gratitude. Feelings cannot be required because they are not wholly subject to rational control. However, Roslyn Weiss calls our attention to mental health professionals who teach individuals not only how to control their feelings but how to change their feelings when given circumstances arise (Weiss, 1985, p. 494). Adult children who have been given benefits from their parents voluntarily, intentionally, benevolently, and in a noncoercive manner should cultivate the attitude of appreciation for these benefits and appreciation and goodwill for their parents.

The gratitude account of filial obligations holds then that the more parents cared about, benefitted, and sacrificed for their children, the greater the responsibility of children to cultivate attitudes of gratitude. We must remember for all cases that the strength of the obligation depends on whether parents met the minimum or whether they went to great lengths. If parents neglected, deprived, or abused their children, these children would not have any filial obligations according to this account.

If one has an obligation to cultivate attitudes of gratitude, what does this mean for the kinds of actions that gratitude would require? The actions required are those that demonstrate the possession of appreciation and goodwill. While gratitude does not require repayments in kind or degree, the types of benefits provided to the children, whether biological, physical, monetary, emotional, and/or intellectual, will most probably shape the form of their gratitude response. We would certainly think the children will have obligations of caregiving and decision making for their parents. What kinds and what amount of caregiving gratitude commits adult children to is really impossible to state at the level of theory. These cannot be specified because they will be context-dependent for the society and for a particular circumstance.

It is disappointing that this conceptual grounding has not yielded a result with more specific implications for long-term care decision making. However, this may in fact not be a "fault" of the argument. Instead, gratitude's apparent lack of specification may rightly reflect the complexity and ambiguity of the subject matter of filial obligations as adult children actually experience and respond to them.

It may at first seem that with the gratitude account filial obligations

are absolute (i.e., without exception or limit in practice). Thus understood, filial obligations would commit adult children to tremendous,
eventually unrealistic, and possibly self-destructive levels of care. Neither of these assumptions is correct for the account presented here. Gratitude obligations are neither absolute nor unlimited. As Daniel Callahan
has said, "That the moral claim made upon them (caregivers) may seem
a justifiable one in many respects does not mean that it will be endurable; that it is endurable does not mean that it is justifiable" (Callahan, 1988, p. 323).

A central theme of this book is that obligations to provide long-term
care by family members are limited. Gratitude-based obligations do not
inherently override all other obligations. They may be viewed as *prima
facie* obligations or obligations that ought to be fulfilled unless meeting
them would conflict with other important obligations of similar strin-
gency, e.g., of adult children to their own spouses and children. The gratitude account though does not tell us in theory what we ought to do
when we have competing obligations, even competing obligations of
gratitude. Ross says that we can only determine the rightness of acts by
determining for an agent in a certain circumstance which act has the
"greatest balance of *prima facie* rightness ... over *prima facie* wrong-
ness." He has, however, no theoretical strategy for how these aspects
are to be compared (Ross, 1930, pp. 41 and 42; Brody, 1988, pp. 96
and 97).

These conflicts must be negotiated in the long-term care decision
making process itself. This negotiation can usefully be structured by the
following conceptual considerations. For adult children there may be
competing obligations to other, special loved ones, such as to minor children. In case of minor children, obligations are thought to flow forward
(Sidgwick, 1962). In other words, when obligations to parents and to
children are in conflict, the obligations to the younger generation sometimes justifiably override those of filial obligations. For long-term care
decision making, this means that in situations where obligations to elderly parents and to young children conflict, adult children may justifiably look to formal systems of support rather than providing personal
caregiving or to social programs of financial assistance rather than
spending all the family resources for formal support. The professional
should help the family see such measures not as moral failures, for which
they might feel guilt, but as morally appropriate and even morally required actions. The policy implications of this analysis are clear and

urgent: more, not less, social resources should be allocated for quality long-term care programs and institutions in order to support families who are faced with these difficult choices.

We should specify that the situation envisioned above included the additional assumption that the needs of the elderly and those of the young children were roughly proportionate. Certainly, needs outweigh requests, and an elderly parent who has basic life-threatening needs may have a greater claim on the resources of the adult child than young children have on the parent's resources when the children request life-enhancing benefits, for example, ballet lessons or summer camp. The duties to elderly parents may not always override those to young children, and a constant moral balancing is required.

Similar to the limitation of spousal obligations of care giving, the extent of caregiving may be limited or overridden by the goals and projects of the caregiver (Jecker, Chap. 8) or *prima facie* duties to self. The film "Like Water for Chocolate" portrays a particular family in Mexico in which the tradition was that the youngest daughter in a family not marry and take care of her mother until her mother's death. This sacrifice was considered obligatory on the daughter's part by the mother. The mother in the film treated her youngest daughter in a callous manner and even in an emotionally cruel way. Because of the context of this tradition, ought the girl not marry and take care of the mother in old age? The answer to this is no.

According to the gratitude account, surely no filial duties were due from this youngest daughter. But what if the mother had treated the girl well? Would gratitude duties be owed? According to this analysis, yes. This daughter may have had some responsibility to care for her mother, but not to meet every obligation that her parent demanded. The youngest daughter had a right to pursue her own projects, to exercise her personal freedom, and to live with integrity (Williams, 1988, pp. 108–118). The obligation to herself may justifiably override this family tradition. The broader culture of Mexico, moreover, accepts that young women should be able to marry if they wish, that children should take care of their parents, and that the two are not mutually exclusive. In fact, the demands placed on this daughter would generally be considered unreasonable in the broader Mexican culture. The girl may have a responsibility to care for her mother, but it does not override all other obligations, such as those to self and others.

Additionally, any other child, male or female, in a family may have gratitude obligations as well. Daughters outnumber sons as caregivers three to one. Women working full time are four times as likely to be primary caregivers to the elderly as are working men (Older Women's League, 1989, p. 3). Men, though, are assuming greater caregiving responsibilities. For those men who are caregivers, there are no significant differences in the amount of time spent caregiving between male and female caregivers. However, the division of caregiving labor is still very gender-based. Men usually help with transportation, home repairs, and financial management, rather than with personal care (Older Women's League, 1989, p. 4). These kinds of caregiving are less emotionally and often less physically demanding than personal caregiving. Therefore, the responsibilities are still disproportionately placed upon women.

The implications for long-term care decision making seem plain. Professionals ought to help families see that ethically the role of primary, personal caregiver should not be ascribed "automatically" to daughters and daughters-in-law. Furthermore, although it is recognized that in practice the role of *primary* caregiver may appropriately be assumed by or given to one particular child, an ethical analysis of filial responsibility does not support a long-term care model that ascribes caregiving to a sole child. (Though it is the case that other children may not have obligations of gratitude because parents failed to provide benefits, voluntarily and benevolently, for the sake of the child.) Even if one child is designated and accepts the role of primary caregiver or decision maker, this does not absolve other children from filial obligations. Professionals justifiably should encourage children to share responsibility for parents' care in the long-term care decision-making process. Future models of long-term care planning ought to include discussions of how caregiving and decision making will be and ought to be shared among all adult children in the family who have obligations of gratitude.

Conclusion

It is well recognized in the gerontological literature that the history of relationship between an elder and the adult children who are caregivers is crucial to understanding the sense of satisfaction and stress that caregivers experience (Brody, 1984). The concept of gratitude as the basis of filial obligations helps to identify the ethical dimensions of that history. The central lesson of this chapter is that if certain aspects of the parent-child relationship are present, adult children will have obligations of gratitude which include the obligation to cultivate the moral attitudes of appreciation and goodwill toward the parent. Most likely, fulfilling filial gratitude obligations will include caregiving or a central role in long-term care decision making concerning the health of the parent. Thus, acknowledgement of gratitude-based obligations should be part of practice and planning.

In long-term care practice, it is important for professionals, elders, and family members to understand that most adult children have some level of obligation that requires them to help with the care of their parents. However, filial obligations must be met by all the adult children who have such responsibilities and not only by daughters and daughters-in-law. Also, as seen above, these obligations are neither unlimited nor absolute. Guidelines to structure negotiation of cases of conflicting obligations have been identified and have practical implications. Professionals need to recognize that in some circumstances it may be justifiable for adult children to meet their filial obligations in severely limited ways, if at all. A gratitude-based understanding of filial obligations also helps the professional to appreciate that gratitude is not only something experienced by the child. Caregiving motivated by gratitude is also experienced as such by the elder. Caregivers are asked to provide care to a more disabled population for a longer period of time than ever before in our history. Older care recipients who recognize this may be very supportive and understanding of the balancing of filial obligations with other special moral obligations. The mutuality of gratitude is a key practice concept.

Conversely, it is also important for professionals to recognize that in families where parents failed child caring obligations or did not provide benefits to children voluntarily and benevolently, children do not have filial obligations (though this does not preclude them from caregiving but merely states that caregiving is not required).

Finally, I have argued that filial obligations of caregiving exist for most people. Public policy needs to focus on making it easier for individuals to meet their obligations to parents. One current irony of formal service provision is the penalty that some families face if they do provide assistance, i.e., discharge their obligations of gratitude as a matter of course. Under Social Security, recipients of supplemental security income receive a lesser amount if they move into the household of an adult child, an option that a grateful child may well be willing to offer. In such situations, an adult child may need to stop working to care for a parent and yet not be able to afford the loss of income. Likewise, the design of some programs results in restricted income and service benefits for those families involved in caring for older parents and, in fact, penalizes them for taking on caregiving responsibilities. The Family and Medical Leave Act, recently enacted in the United States, provides job protection for adult children caregivers (among others), but the leave is without pay and for a very limited amount of time. Planning and policy should be reconsidered so that they support—but do not exploit—gratitude-based filial obligations. Incentives and rewards for family support should be reconsidered, perhaps via tax credits and direct payment to family caregivers. Any new health care plan should include funding for home health care, respite care, and adult day care centers. These are the policy issues that the gratitude account of filial obligations raises that must be addressed concerning filial responsibility for long-term care decision making within the family.

REFERENCES

Aristotle. (1941). Nicomachean ethics. In Richard McKeon (ed.), *The Basic Works of Aristotle*, Bk. V, ch. 5. New York: Random House.

Becker, L.C. (1986). *Reciprocity*. London: Routledge & Kegan Paul.

Berger, F.R. (1985). Gratitude. *Ethics*, 95: 298–309.

Blackstone. (1856). *Commentaries on the Laws of England, Vol. 1, Book 1, ch. 16, sect. 1*. Philadelphia. J. B. Lippincott.

Brody, B.A. (1988). *Life and Death Decision-Making*. New York: Oxford University Press.

Brody, E.M. (1984). What should adult children do for elderly parents? Opinions and preferences of three generations of women. *Journal of Gerontology*, 39: 736–746.

Callahan, D. (1985). What do children owe elderly parents? *Hastings Center Report*, 15: 32–37.

Callahan, D. (1988). Families as caregivers: The limits of morality. *Archives of Physical Medicine Rehabilitation*, 69: 323–328.

Card, C. (1988). Gratitude and Obligation. *American Philosophical Quarterly*, 25: 115–127.

Christiansen, D. (1987). Ethical guidelines for assisting the elderly. *America*, 156: 72–75.

Goodin, R.E. (1985). *Protecting the Vulnerable: A Reanalysis of Our Social Responsibilities*. Chicago: University of Chicago Press.

Kant, I. (1797). Doctrine of virtues, Pt. II. In *The Metaphysics of Morals,* trans. M. Gregor, pp. 181–279. New York: Cambridge University Press, reprint 1991.

Lewin, T. (1989). Ailing parent: Women's burden grows. The *New York Times,* November 13, A1, p. 13.

Older Women's League. (1989). *Failing America's Caregivers: A Status Report on Women Who Care.* Washington, D.C.: Older Women's League.

Ross, D.W. (1930). *The Right and the Good.* Oxford: Clarendon Press.

Sidgwick, H. (1962). *The Methods of Ethics.* Chicago: University of Chicago Press.

Simmons, A.J. (1979). *Moral Principles and Political Obligations.* Princeton, N.J.: Princeton University Press.

Weiss, R. (1985). The moral and social dimensions of gratitude. *Southern Journal of Philosophy, 23:* 491–501.

Williams, B. (1988). A critique of utilitarianism. In J.J.C. Smart and B. Williams (eds.), *Utilitarianism: For and Against,* pp. 77–155. New York: Cambridge University Press.

CHAPTER TEN

Conflicting Interests in Long-Term Care
Decision Making: Acknowledging, Dissolving, and
Resolving Conflicts

John D. Arras

The Patient-Centered Moral Framework of Acute Care Medicine

Traditional medical ethics exhibits a nearly exclusive concern for the physician-patient relationship. In contrast to other ethical stances, such as utilitarianism or perfectionism, the Hippocratic tradition enshrines the health and welfare of the patient as the doctor's sole proper concern (Levinsky, 1984). The contemporary, autonomy-driven models of medical ethics have likewise focused upon the desires and interests of the patient. Developed largely in a context of acute-care medicine, the contractualist model has inherited the patient-centered emphasis of the ancient Hippocratic tradition (Veatch, 1972). The choices that doctors and patients make, however, do not take place in a social vacuum. The interests of others, such as family members, other patients in the unit, future patients, and those currently lacking access to care, can be significantly affected by decisions to pursue the best interests of some patients. When physicians order a new drug that is slightly more effective but extraordinarily more expensive than the standard brand, they may be placing a heavy burden on the family's budget. When neonatologists unilaterally decide to prolong, by means of hyperalimentation, the life of a child doomed from birth with inoperable short gut syndrome, they often consign the parents to lives of stress and sorrow until the child eventually succumbs.

While these sorts of interests and burdens would obviously matter a great deal in other nonmedical contexts and figure prominently in decision making there, they tend not to count in the moral context of acute-care medicine. In the modern hospital, the "doctor's workshop," medical concerns take priority over nonmedical values, such as expense or social burdens to families or society, and the interests of present patients take priority over the interests of other parties (Hardwig, 1990).

When it is suggested that such an "extraneous" interest might be influencing decisions made on behalf of a patient, such that the "best interests" of the patient might be sacrificed or attenuated, a red flag immediately looms: this, we say, is a "conflict of interest." Examples easily come to mind. A young couple anxious to have a "normal baby" suddenly refuse necessary surgery for their child born with a chromosomal disorder such as Down syndrome and duodenal atresia. The grown children of an abusive, mildly demented parent with a good chance for meaningful quality of life urge doctors to "let nature take its course" rather than aggressively treat pneumonia. A physician-entrepreneur acquires ownership of a diagnostic laboratory to which he regularly refers all of his patients.

Within the acute-care setting, the customary response to perceived conflicts of interest is to disqualify the decision maker. Rather than simply stating a fact, namely, that a discordance exists between the respective interests of the patient and decision maker, the invocation of these words usually expresses a moral conclusion. Indeed, to say of a decision maker that he or she has a conflict of interest is to say, in effect, that their decision is *tainted* and, thus, that someone else should make the decision.

As in legal or political settings, then, the notion of conflict of interest tends to function in the acute-care environment as a kind of "threshold concept," that is, as a concept that determines, in an all or nothing fashion, whether someone is fit or qualified for the role of decision maker (Buchanan and Brock, 1989). Just as the concept of "decision-making capacity" *qualifies* someone as a decision maker, so the concept of "conflict of interest" *disqualifies* someone for this same role. Thus, we say that the parents of the Down syndrome child should bow to the wishes of a *guardian ad litem,* that the grown children of the abusive parent should either consent to treatment or the doctors should do so for them, and that the physician-entrepreneur should divest himself of his financial interest in the laboratory.

Decision makers with conflicts of interest are usually disqualified for one or another of two related reasons. In some cases, the conflict might prevent someone from fairly and adequately assessing the patient's preferences or best interest. Thus, the physician-entrepreneur can be expected to be sorely tempted to place his own financial interests above those of his patients. In other cases, the would-be surrogate's conflicting interests are judged to have no legitimate moral weight in the circumstances. Even though physicians and hospital administrators might be sympathetic to the couple seeking a "normal baby," this desire is given no moral weight when placed on the scale opposite the child's interest in and ability to live a life not disproportionately burdened by Down syndrome.

In the context of acute-care medicine, then, a highly idealized picture of decision making emerges, a parallel to George Agich's concept of "ideal" autonomy, described in Chapter 6. Whoever is charged with making decisions for ill and impaired patients, whether it be physicians or involved family or friends, they are expected to decide solely on the ground of the patient's desires or best interests. This picture tends to exclude in principle any and all interests on the part of physicians and family that might conflict with those of the patient. The rationale for this wholesale exclusion of conflicting interests appears to be a complex amalgam of ethical principle and history.

On the one hand, a defender of this patient-centered moral framework could point to the importance of health needs vis-à-vis other kinds of needs. The patient-centered framework can also be seen as a necessary shield for persons whose autonomy, voice, and independence have been seriously eroded by illness. Patients whose very lives, health, identity, and future are under siege are extremely vulnerable; they need not only the doctor's care but the doctor's protection as well. The last thing that many seriously ill patients need during their time of personal crisis and disorientation is a more robust sensitivity to the needs of others.

Historical factors may also figure in the explanation and justification of an unrelentingly patient-centered perspective. The traditional Hippocratic model of the physician-patient relationship, defined by the physician's exclusive fiduciary relationship to the patient, was developed well before the advent of scientific medicine, the ensuing explosion of chronic illness, and the modern hospital. In previous eras physicians could profess and act on their duty of exclusive fidelity to the patient without thereby placing undue burdens on the family or other caregivers.

The patient centeredness of the traditional Hippocratic ethical framework was no doubt reinforced by the rise of the modern, acute-care hospital. Because patients came to them on their own turf, doctors practicing in acute-care settings had much greater success in establishing an exclusively patient-centered moral environment. And since acute-care medicine, rather than either family medicine or home care, came to symbolize all the power, prestige, and promise of "modern medicine," it is no wonder that the moral framework elaborated in this setting should have achieved hegemony over alternative ethical models developed in various medical "backwaters," such as long-term care.

Things are not quite this simple, however, even in the acute-care setting. Although peremptory dismissal is the usual response to conflicts of interest on the part of decision makers, there is another, more nuanced and complicated use of the phrase that tends to replicate another important feature of the concept of decision-making capacity. Just as this latter notion can express the bottom line of a complicated process of reasoning, involving the weighing and balancing of competing values, so the notion of "conflict of interest" can also, on occasion, express a kind of "all things considered judgment." In this sense, to disqualify someone as having a conflict of interest could mean not that any and all conflicts automatically disqualify a decision maker, but rather that this particular conflict is too serious, the projected harm to the patient too great, to allow this person to decide. This suggests, again, taking our cue from the logic of competency judgments, that conflict of interest determinations are sometimes aligned on a "sliding scale" of seriousness and risk (Drane, 1985).

Examples of this phenomenon abound in the discharge-planning process that bridges the gap between acute and long-term care. Rosalie Kane and Arthur Caplan (1990, p. 112) cite the case of an elderly patient who, while strongly bonded to caretaking family members, appeared to be receiving substandard or possibly even somewhat "neglectful" care at home. The patient lacked decision-making capacity, yet exhibited a vehement and unambiguous desire to return home. This plea disconcerted the patient's case manager, who was not only worried about the low quality of care at home but also about the family's rather unseemly financial interest in keeping the patient's monthly check for themselves.

In such a case there may well be a bona fide conflict of interest between the family and the patient. If the family truly had the patient's best *medical* interests in mind, they would have either given the patient better home care or placed her in a nursing home. Still, it might be best "all things considered" for the discharge planners to send the patient home. She may continue to receive a worrisomely low quality of care, but this disadvantage may be sufficiently offset by the patient's keen desire to return to the bosom of her trusted family where she feels most alive and at home, perhaps in pursuit of independence in the rich sense provided for this term in Chapter 7 by Bart Collopy. The nursing home might provide this patient better nursing care and medical monitoring, but those benefits might be outweighed by a spirit-breaking exile from hearth and home. In Collopy's (Chap. 7) terms, the nursing home would not, all things considered, be safe.

A central theme of this volume is that with this sort of case we reach the outer boundary of the exclusively patient-centered moral framework of acute-care medicine, a boundary where interesting and important questions remain unasked and unanswered. Agich (Chap. 6) and Collopy (Chap. 7) explored such questions, questions that, as Kane (Chap. 5) and Terrie Wetle (Chap. 4) pointed out earlier, confront care providers and families.

In this chapter, this central theme is explored by raising the following kinds of questions: Given their manifest significance and weight, why shouldn't the interests of family and caretaking friends be taken more seriously? Instead of always being subordinated to the patient's health-related interests, instead of being relegated to the status of a mere "cost of doing business" within an overall patient-centered calculus of benefits and burdens, why shouldn't the interests of family and close friends count for something *in their own right*? Indeed, why shouldn't the legitimate interests of caretakers sometimes actually outweigh the interests of the patient? Addressing these questions helps to set the stage for the preventive ethics approach to long-term care decision making discussed in the next chapter.

Beyond the Patient-Centered Framework: The Challenge of Long-Term Care

In contrast to acute-care medicine, the contexts of long-term care fairly bristle with a wide variety of acknowledged interests, many of which conflict. In nursing homes, rehabilitation centers, and private homes the conflicts are so numerous, and the interests of the various parties so obviously pressing and legitimate, that the idealized, acute-care conception of the disinterested decision maker cannot be seriously maintained, even as a useful fiction.

In nursing homes and rehabilitation centers, many of the most vexing ethical problems have to do not with the "big ticket" life and death dilemmas, but rather with the small-scale conflicts of everyday life (Kane and Caplan, 1990), a theme emphasized in this volume by Agich (Chap. 6) and Collopy (Chap. 7). Instead of occupying discrete spatial units of highly focused care within the "doctor's workshop," residents of nursing homes and other long-term care facilities actually live and cohabit in these institutions. In these "home-like" spaces, each resident's desires, interests, and actions can impact directly on the interests and legitimate expectations of others. Patients who wander into others' rooms, make loud noises, or refuse to bathe have a direct impact on the quality of life of other residents and the staff. An exclusively autonomy-driven ethic fails to acknowledge the obvious point that the nursing home is *their* home too.

The patient-centered ethical framework of acute-care medicine is even less appropriate in the context of private homes, the venue of long-term home care. Here the best interests of the patient often conflict with the desires, needs, and interests of other family members (Collopy, Dubler, and Zuckerman, 1990). Consider the case of Mr. O'Brien, an elderly hospitalized alcoholic whose care at home had begun to impose insupportable demands upon his devoted daughter, who cared for him in his apartment while also juggling the needs of her husband and small children. The patient, viewed by the staff as an extraordinarily mean-spirited and demanding person, was no doubt near dying from multiple medical problems and wanted above all else to go home. The medical team felt that his needs were so enormous that he would be better cared for in a nursing home, but they also worried about the burdens that granting the patient's wish would impose on his daughter. This woman was caught between the competing demands of her own family, including several children, and those of her father. Her brother, who had long ago given up on their neglectful and rancorous father, confided to the doctors that his sister had told him that she had reached the limit of her endurance, but he warned that she was simply incapable of ever saying "no" to her father, whom she adored. Should the physicians act exclusively as agents of the patient's autonomous, if selfish, desires, or should they be equally if not more concerned with the imposition of unfair burdens upon a devoted daughter?

Although home care can offer significant benefits to all concerned, especially given the dismal alternatives in most nursing homes and long-term institutions, it can also place extraordinary demands on caregivers. Caring for a loved one with severe Alzheimer's disease, for example, can be an all-consuming task, often eclipsing entirely the caregiver's life beyond the routines of care at home. This potential downside of home care has recently become an even more serious problem with the advent of so-called "high-tech" home care (Arras and Dubler, 1995). Long-term care thus represents a fundamental challenge to the traditional patient-centered ethic associated with acute-care medicine.

In homes and nursing homes, the categorical exclusion of all interests that might potentially conflict with the patient's best interest appears to be manifestly unjust. These others are people too, and any ethic of long-term care must treat them with concern and respect. Although the needs of chronically ill persons are themselves deserving of special attention, and although most family members and caregiving friends no doubt wish to give them a full measure of care, there are limits that a responsible ethic of long-term care must observe (Blustein, 1993; Hardwig, 1990; Nelson, 1992). At the very least, caregivers must not be forced to relinquish their legitimate claims to have a life apart from the demands of caring. Mr. O'Brien's daughter may indeed have interests weighty enough to eclipse her father's single-minded desire to return home. The realities of long-term care thus highlight a fact that should have been obvious to us even in the context of acute-care medicine: there are potentially conflicting interests everywhere in long-term care decision making and in everyone, including physicians, nursing home administrators, and loving family members.

The challenge for an ethic of long-term care, then, is not to expunge these conflicting interests, a move that would often result in serious injustice to affected parties, but rather to learn how best to strike an appropriate balance among them and attempt to prevent ethical conflicts those interests might engender (McCullough et al., Chap. 11). As Nancy Dubler has persuasively argued elsewhere (1990, p. 159; Collopy, Dubler, and Zuckerman, 1990; see also Moody, 1992), instead of enshrining the patient's best interest as the overriding goal of long-term care, viewing all conflicting interests as being somehow tainted, we must develop an alternative model based upon notions of fairness, accommodation, compromise, and negotiation. Such an alternative model would clarify the kinds of patient interests that might be ethically compromised and the kinds of caregiver interests that might, on occasion, override the best interests of patients.

Refining the Ethic of Accommodation

The interests of patients, family members, and care providers fall across a very broad spectrum, ranging from the most serious to the merely trivial, selfish, or harmful. It goes without saying that patients have important interests that require protection and care. At the top of this list are interests in life itself, the restoration of function, freedom from pain and suffering, and the nurturing presence of loved ones. At the other extreme, rarely mentioned in the lore of acute-care medicine, are interests or preferences that might be judged selfish, spiteful, or harmful to both self and others.

Consider in this connection the case of L.R., a 70-year-old woman in need of serious rehabilitation therapy (Ackerman and Strong, 1989, p. 12). Although her physicians and therapists see no physical reason why she cannot improve her range of function, L.R. refuses therapy, apparently because she is quite comfortable with her present home situation in which her increasingly beleaguered husband does all the cooking and housework for her. The couple's daughter fears that her father cannot sustain this workload much longer and has begun looking into a nursing home placement for her mother. L.R. wishes above all else to remain at home, but she refuses to permit the very treatment that will allow her to assume more household responsibilities, relieve her husband of his crushing burden, and thus forestall placement in a nursing home. For his part, the husband has no strong opinion about the nursing home option and appears willing to leave the decision up to his daughter. The case poses the question of whether L.R.'s caregivers should honor at face value her competent refusal of rehabilitative interventions or whether they should exert their influence upon her to alter her apparently short-sighted, self-defeating, and selfish refusal to do more on her own behalf.

The interests of family members and other surrogates exhibit the same complex structure. Some families are simply dysfunctional and ill-equipped for the role of decision maker. Their members may be aloof, disconnected from the patient, squeamish about making difficult decisions, selfish, irresponsible, vindictive, irrational, childish, or simply incapable of comprehending the facts or alternatives. At the other end of the spectrum, some families are heroic and saintly. They show a single-minded, unstinting devotion to the care of a loved one, self-consciously and freely choosing to subordinate their entire lives to the well-being of a child, spouse, or parent. In between these extremes, there are the vast majority of families that simply want to "do the right thing" for their loved ones. Indeed, I would argue that most families have a powerful interest in providing loving, personalized care to their members. When they fail to do so, the failure is more than likely due to the inadequacies of our health care "system" and social supports than to any demonstrable conflict of interest (Noddings, 1995; Wilson, Chap. 3).

Nevertheless, there are limits to what can or should be expected from family members or caregiving friends. When a parent has spent a lifetime being neglectful and abusive, his children may have a legitimate interest in being free of him. (Mr. O'Brien's son certainly has no remaining moral obligation to care at home for his misanthropic and alcoholic father.) Or the demands of care may be so great in terms of emotional drain, financial expense, and time that the caregiver, usually a woman, ceases to have a life of her own (Wilson, Chap. 3). Such caregivers have a legitimate, justice-based interest in having a life apart from caring for others (Jecker, Chap. 8).

In addition to their interests in choosing their own relationships and pursuing their own projects, family members are enmeshed in complicated webs of duties, some of which may compromise others. As moral agents committed to more than one person at a time, family members have an important interest in achieving some sort of reasonable balance among these conflicting duties.

Sarah Brakman and Nancy Jecker explored some strategies for balancing interests in the previous two chapters. Here I want to take up a suggestion made elsewhere by Jecker (1993) that the family economy might profitably be conceived as a kind of "commons" from which each is entitled to withdraw only his or her "fair share" of care. The nature and magnitude of each person's share will, of course, depend crucially upon the particularities of each family's resources, relationships, and history. We cannot tell whether someone is placing undue strain on the family commons simply by referring to their formal role or status in the family (for example, as father or daughter) or by the amount of time others must devote to his or her care. Everything will depend upon the meaning that the particular caring enterprise has for all of the involved parties.

Nevertheless, there is a limit to what any family commons can dispense to one member in terms of time, energy, and attention, another central theme of this volume (Brakman, Chap. 9; Jecker, Chap. 8; Mc-Cullough et al., Chap. 11). When that threshold is crossed, the neglect of the rightful expectations of the others becomes a matter of justice. Thus, while Mr. O'Brien's daughter had an interest in caring for her father, she also had important obligations to her own husband and children. Although Mr. O'Brien may still possibly have had some sort of tenuous moral claim on his daughter's time and attention—a point that his son would contest—Mr. O'Brien certainly has no right to her nearly exclusive concern at the expense of her own needs and those of her family.

Finally, family members might also have a legitimate stake in defending the family as a unit. Although the family is often disparaged today—quite accurately, I'm afraid—as a hothouse of dysfunctionality, for many the family still serves as a unique source of intimacy and nurturance in their lives, as a buffer between the individual and the impersonal forces of market and state. To the extent that the burdens of providing long-term care can strain existing family ties, transforming a "haven in a heartless world" into a crucible of need, stress, and fatigue, family members may have a legitimate interest in lessening that burden so as to maintain the integrity of their intimate connections (Nelson and Nelson, in press, 1995).

Thus, our stereotypical picture of conflicts of interest, pitting "sacred" patient interests in life against "profane" family interests in money or irresponsible freedom, leaves out the possibilities at the other end of these respective spectrums of interest (L.R.'s selfish refusal of rehabilitation versus her husband's justice-based claims to a shared workload) and the entire gray area in between these poles. With a more complex understanding of the nature of the various interests at stake in long-term care now in hand, we can proceed to offer some observations regarding their moral assessment.

Assessing Conflicting Interests

In spite of its shortcomings in the context of long-term care, the standard patient-centered moral framework may still have much to contribute, if not as a comprehensive moral standard then at least as the basis of a moral presumption that must be overcome. It still makes good sense, I believe, to begin our assessment of conflicting interests with a presumption in favor of attempting to foster and honor the autonomous choices or best interests of elders, even in a chronic care setting, particularly with reference to what Agich described as nodal and interstitial long-term care decisions in Chapter 6.

This presumption is based upon three considerations. First, more often than not, the patient's interests will be urgent and weighty: the preservation of life, the restoration of healthy function, the alleviation of pain and suffering, and return to the bosom of family life. Even if other family members or caregiving friends have interests in conflict with these, their interests will usually be neither as pressing nor as weighty as the patient's. Second, it will be difficult in practice to strike a fair balance between the interests of patients, whose strength and voice may have been sapped by chronic disease and disability, and the interests of other parties. Given the ease with which the well might overpower or discount the legitimate interests of the chronically ill, it makes sense to erect a patient-oriented presumption in order to better approximate just and fair resolutions of competing claims. Finally, it is reasonable to expect health-related institutions and programs, such as hospitals, nursing homes, and home care, to focus on what they know best: how to foster the health and welfare of the individual patient. While it would be nice if society could somehow provide us with a forum and an authority for weighing and balancing the wide variety of conflicting interests that pervade long-term care, there is no reason to think that health care providers have any special insight or skill regarding the fair resolution of such conflicts.

Given the countervailing claims of others based upon standards of fairness and justice, however, this presumption in favor of the patient's autonomous wishes and best interest remains eminently rebuttable. We come, then, to the crucial question: when may the patient's wishes or interests be set aside in favor of the conflicting interests of others?

A central theme of this volume is that no handy rule or algorithm will guide us through this moral thicket. Too much depends upon the particularities of each case: the values and expectations of the various parties, the history of their tangled relationships, the consequent meaning of events and choices to different people, the setting, and so on.

Still, particular decisions can be roughly arranged along two related sliding scales: the less serious or more ethically questionable the patient's choices or interests and the stronger the family's claims, the more justifiable it will be to overturn the usual presumption in favor of the patient. Thus, given the selfish and ultimately self-defeating nature of L.R.'s interest in refusing rehabilitation therapy to maintain her indolent life style, her husband's important interests in maintaining his own health and sanity, as well as his interest in a fair allocation of burdens at home, tip the scales in his favor. At the very least, her health care providers are ethically justified in discounting her own firmly stated desires and attempting to argue strongly with her in favor of more rehabilitative therapy; at most, they are entitled to throw their considerable weight behind the daughter's attempt to place her mother in a nursing home. Likewise, even though Mr. O'Brien's fervent wish to return home to be cared for by his devoted daughter reflects a very significant interest ordinarily deserving of our respect, his failure even to consider her own interests and competing responsibilities to her own family constitutes a kind of moral "trespass" on the commons of family care. There is only so much to go around, and he has demanded much more than his fair share.

This legitimation of balancing conflicting interests among patients and family raises an important question bearing on the *kinds* of patient interests that might be ethically subordinated to those of other family members. One might be tempted to respond that it is one thing to discount unjust incursions into the family commons, arguing that the patient has no legitimate interest in unlimited caring on the part of family, but quite another to subordinate the patient's interests in life or health to the family's nonmedical concerns. This response would thus claim, for example, that family members who do most of the actual work associated with home care are thereby ethically justified in setting limits upon a patient's demands, while the families of nursing home or rehabilitation patients should not be allowed to act on conflicts of interest, especially when the latter impinge upon the patient's life or health. In such cases, it is argued, the patient-centered ethic should prevail.

Although this limitation on the kinds of patient interests that will be permitted on our sliding scale is perhaps intuitively attractive, I believe that this position is also best formulated as a presumption rather than as an absolute prohibition. In the first place, we must acknowledge that the resolution of some conflicts over the family commons will predictably have adverse effects upon the health or life expectancy of some chronically ill patients. When an exhausted family finally decides to place a loved one in a nursing home, a number of factors may conspire to depress the patient and even to shorten the patient's life. So we already allow some conflicts to be resolved by placing patients' interests in health or life on our sliding scale. Secondly, some chronically ill patients may be so dramatically damaged that they arguably cease to have any remaining interest in further care or in being kept alive. Consider, for example, residents of chronic care facilities who are in a persistent vegetative state (PVS). Such patients have no capacity for conscious life, they can no longer interact with their environment, and they therefore lack the capacity to be benefitted or harmed by medical treatment or bedside caring. Assuming that a particular PVS patient had not previously expressed a desire to be maintained in such a state, a desire that may not command much respect in any case due to considerations of social justice, I contend that just about any kind of family burden, financial or emotional, incurred by the maintenance of such a patient would suffice to justify the termination of treatment and the patient's biological life (Arras, 1991).

Patients who are not in a PVS yet manifest extreme dementia may constitute a second category wherein conflicting family interests may legitimately be placed on the scale alongside the patient's interest in health or extended life. Such patients, notwithstanding their inability to recognize or interact with others, may nevertheless have an interest in securing pleasurable sensations or avoiding noxious stimuli. We may want to argue in such extreme cases, though we cannot pursue the argument here, that such an attenuated set of interests might be legitimately sacrificed to important conflicting family interests, including an interest in avoiding serious financial or emotional hardship (Arras, 1988; Dresser and Robertson, 1989). Although I believe that a strong case could be made for the interpersonal balancing of these kinds of interests, great care would have to be exercised to avoid falling headlong down the slippery slope of discrimination and neglect of demented patients who retain serious interests in continued care and prolonged life.

Steps toward the Dissolution and Resolution of Conflicting Interests in Long-Term Care

It is one thing to grant on the level of theory that the chronically ill patient's interests may sometimes be legitimately outweighed by the competing interests of others; it is quite another to devise fair procedures and practical strategies for implementing our notions of the family commons and caring within the bounds of justice.

Before we settle down to the difficult, confusing, and dangerous business of suggesting practical mechanisms for assessing the conflicting interests of patients and families, we should first investigate the extent to which such conflicts might be attenuated or dissolved altogether through what might be called a "social fix." Many conflicts between the respective interests of patients and families stem, as Nancy Wilson showed in Chapter 3, from inadequate social and psychological supports (for example, undesirable nursing homes, spend down requirements, lack of intermediate institutions between the hospital and home, or lack of respite care to relieve family caregivers) that have deep roots in the history described at the beginning of this volume by Martha Holstein and Thomas Cole. Our first reaction as a society should be to provide the missing supports rather than contemplate violations of the patient's interests (Minow, 1990, pp. 334, 339; Noddings, in press 1995; Asch, 1990, pp. 113–120). When confronted by conflicting interests, we need to expand our circle of awareness beyond the demands of individual patients and the limitations of individual caregivers to encompass a perspective emphasizing social duties and social supports for caregivers and families. As we observed above, most caregivers and families sincerely wish to do the right thing, that is, to do what they can, within reason, to provide loving care. Society should make every reasonable effort to help them do this. Above all, we should not stigmatize families for succumbing to pressures created in the first place by societal neglect.

Apart from the provision of necessary services, health care providers can do much to attenuate excessive pressures on caregivers, especially in the home care setting, by recognizing the fluctuating nature both of the burdens of caring and of the capacities of caregivers to endure. Often families who take chronically ill loved ones home from the hospital have no realistic notion of just how demanding their care will be. In other cases, a care plan that begins as a manageable enterprise, for example, converting a dining room into a bedroom for a frail parent to move in with her son and his family, may become more and more onerous due to the patient's worsening condition until the family's emotional resources have been stretched to the breaking point. In either sort of case, families will often experience feelings of failure and guilt for having "given up." Health care providers should alert family caregivers to the possibility of future strains upon the family commons and reassure them that the initial "caregiving contract" will be subject to continuous revision in the light of the patient's changing prognosis or increasing burdens upon the family. This is a key element of the preventive ethics approach to long-term care decision making described in the next chapter.

In the end, however, we must acknowledge that not all conflicts are amenable to dissolution through the provision of social supports or renegotiable treatment plans. In some cases, the source of a family's conflicting interests is due to the kind of emotional burnout that no amount of supplementary services could prevent; in many other cases, however, the needed social supports simply do not materialize. What practical steps can then be taken to ameliorate or resolve such conflicts? More specifically (and problematically), how can we practically implement our theoretical conclusion that the family's interests should count and sometimes even outweigh the interests of patients in long-term care?

We can begin by noting that decisional authority should be linked to the respective stakes of the involved parties. Judged against this standard, overburdened or abused caregivers at home may have a unilateral moral entitlement to set limits on the amount of caring they are required to do and even, in extreme cases, to deny a patient access to their home. It is, after all, *their* home too. Mr. O'Brien's daughter, for example, has a perfect right to insist, both on her own behalf and on that of her family, that her father receive all or part of his care at home from someone else; and L.R.'s husband is morally entitled to insist that his wife either cooperate with rehabilitation or move to a nursing home.

While the unilateral invocation of rights within the family commons may mark the appropriate resolution of some extreme conflicts in home care, the vast majority of cases are more nuanced and call for more subtle modes of resolution. Here the usual bioethical focus on the conflicting rights and interests of individuals may be less appropriate and helpful than a more family-centered ethical framework that views each of the contesting parties, not as a self-contained atom, but rather as a person who is in large part defined and sustained by family bonds. Here the best interests of each usually intersect on some level with the best interests of the others.

The task in this kind of moral setting is to devise, implement, and nurture deliberative processes that enhance communication, empathy, and mutual understanding within a family. Contrary to the "win/lose" orientation of contemporary bioethics, which is constantly asking "who should decide?"—as though finding a single designated decider were the holy grail of good ethics—a more appropriate approach to conflict in this setting would set out to achieve mutually agreeable solutions among family members through the careful articulation of interests, respectful and empathetic listening, creative efforts to "reframe" the question, the efficient and creative marshalling of all available resources, and dignified compromise. In pursuit of this more family-centered deliberative process, health care providers and case managers would do well to borrow a page from lawyers (gasp!), not by focusing on conflicting individual rights in the manner of constitutional and defense attorneys, but rather through the development of a theory and practice of "dispute mediation" (West and Gibson, 1992; Dubler and Marcus, 1994).

Fixing the locus of decisional authority within long-term care institutions is more complex and difficult, both because the family's investment in time and energy is less than in the home setting and because of the patient-centered ethos prevalent in nursing homes, hospitals, and rehabilitation centers. In light of the seriousness of family interests in health care decisions, John Hardwig (1990) has suggested a process of shared decision making among competent patients and affected family. Abandoning entirely the exclusively patient-centered notion of autonomy, Hardwig proposes family conferences authorized to make decisions in the hospital as an ideal procedural mechanism for sorting out and weighing the various conflicting interests. All family members' interests would receive equal consideration, and health interests would be on a par with equally serious interests of other kinds. Decisions would be made through group deliberation.

While Hardwig (1990) deserves credit for calling attention to the moral status of families, I believe that his proposal goes too far in the direction of shared decision making when competent patients are involved. As we saw above, even though an exclusively patient-centered perspective is indeed untenable, there are good reasons to leave a patient-centered *presumption* intact, especially in health care institutions for chronically ill patients. Hardwig's proposal ignores or underestimates both the frailty and vulnerability of these patients, just as it overestimates the varying competence, good faith, and psychological maturity of many families under stress. Given the direct, immediate, and serious impact of many health care decisions on the body and life of the patient and given the natural but unfortunate potential of such family conferences for the subtle coercion of ill or frail patients by more vigorous and more numerous family members, I believe that the ultimate locus of authority in the majority of cases should remain with the competent patient. This means neither that the competent patient has a right to remain isolated in his or her decision-making privacy nor that physicians and family members should not attempt to persuade the patient to acknowledge and duly consider the conflicting interests of others (Blustein, 1993). It simply means that, absent unusual circumstances, the competent patient should retain the presumption of decisional authority. As we noted, however, this remains a presumption that can and should be overcome if and when the patient's interests are relatively slight and the family stands to suffer weighty burdens.

Fixing the locus of decisional authority regarding the care of incompetent patients is an easier matter. There is now a broad consensus that either duly appointed health care proxies or other surrogates drawn from the patient's circle of family and close friends should, barring decisions clearly against the patient's wishes or best interests, be empowered to make decisions. The problem lies in determining the allowable scope of surrogate decisions based on family interests and in deciding whether such decisions should be arrived at through open discussions with health care providers or more obliquely and privately.

Under the regnant consensus, surrogates for incompetent patients are required to base their decisions on patient-centered criteria: namely, either the patient's prior wishes, when available, or best interests. Our theoretical findings with regard to the morals of the family commons would compel a broadening of this mandate to include certain conflicting interests of family members, but the notion of a patient-centered presumption may be useful and appropriate here as well. Incompetent patients are often sicker and more vulnerable than patients able to speak for themselves. To subject them to the sort of "one person, one vote" scenario suggested by the notion of decision-making family conferences may well result all too often in decisions that discriminate against the chronically ill. A presumption that surrogates should focus on patient-centered decision-making criteria, coupled with a willingness to override that presumption when the patient's claims are relatively weak and the family has much to lose, may well strike the right balance between conflicting interests here.

Assuming, then, that the mandate of surrogate decision makers may be broadened on occasion to include consideration of some (possibly conflicting) familial interests, our final question concerns just how open and aboveboard we wish to be about this weighing and balancing within the family commons. One plausible view is that surrogates should be permitted to engage in more family-oriented decision making but should do so quietly, unobtrusively, and obliquely under the rubric of "family discretion." This is to say that as long as the family's decision falls into a morally acceptable gray zone and as long as the patient's legitimate and important interests are not seriously compromised, the family will not be questioned about its choice or compelled to justify its decision to sacrifice some interest of the patient in favor of the family's interest. Family members could simply conclude, "Given all the various factors, we think this is the best decision to make."

This oblique approach to decision making within the family commons would at least have the advantage of imposing minimal stress and guilt on families already faced with difficult and often tragic choices. It is hard enough for families to make perplexing and emotionally freighted decisions without the added burden of having to justify sacrificing the interests of their loved ones—a sacrifice usually mandated by the absence of social supports. Given the overabundant supply of available guilt we all carry with us, it may be asking too much of some surrogate decision makers to confront such conflicts directly and justify putting their own interests, no matter how legitimate and pressing, ahead of the patient's, no matter how trivial, selfish, or wrongheaded.

The major disadvantages of this approach would appear to be its lack of candor and possible encouragement of self-deception on the part of decision makers, on the one hand, and lack of attention to the family's needs for psychological support, on the other. Without the requirement of having to distinguish their own needs from those of the patient, it may be all too easy for surrogates to assume that what is good for them is also good for the patient. And by simply accepting at face value a family's possibly tortured decision, often reached at the conclusion of a long and lonely struggle against adversity, to place its own interests ahead of the patient's, health care providers may simply increase the family's sense of isolation and fail to provide adequate psychological support as family members make what must surely be tragic choices.

An alternative approach would grant surrogates an identical range of authority, while suggesting that decision making within the family commons should openly and frankly confront the problem of trade-offs and compromises among conflicting interests. Proponents of this view might argue that the primary virtue of the oblique approach derives from the status quo's general hostility or indifference to the needs and role of the family. If we had a health care system that cared more about families and the goods that they foster—not to mention a system more sensitive to our society's failure to provide social supports and thus less quick to condemn overburdened family members for harboring conflicting interests—then perhaps a more open dialogue between families and health care providers might be preferable to the relative silence and isolation of family discretion (Minow, 1990, p. 338). According to James Nelson (1992), such an open dialogue could assist families to clarify for themselves the differences between their own interests and those of the patient, and thus could possibly obviate the sort of self-deception encouraged by the oblique approach while still honoring the important interests of both patients and families. Although this more "family friendly" approach is attractive, it would surely require far-reaching changes in public and professional attitudes before it could be practically implemented. Until that time, a more low-key, oblique approach may be the best we can do.

Conclusion

In the context of long-term care decision making, conflicting interests are pervasive, rooted in legitimate claims and expectations, and are usually ineliminable. The highly idealized, patient-centered picture of the doctor-patient relationship that currently governs acute-care settings cannot do justice here. In its place, an alternative model should be developed that takes the interests of patients seriously without denigrating or disqualifying the important interests of others. Whenever possible, medical and social resources should be sought and provided in order to alleviate such conflicts; but in the absence of such a "social fix," just resolutions will depend upon a thorough inventory, accommodation, and balancing of competing interests. The patient-centered perspective should survive this "paradigm shift," but only as a presumption that can and should be rebutted by the presence of serious and legitimate countervailing interests of family members, caregivers, and others. The challenge for the future of long-term care settings is thus to provide a context in which the virtues of both care and justice might flourish.

REFERENCES

Ackerman, T.F., and Strong, C. (1989). *A Casebook of Medical Ethics.* New York: Oxford University Press.

Arras, J.D. (1988). The severely demented, minimally functional patient: An ethical analysis. *Journal of the American Geriatrics Society, 36:* 938–944.

Arras, J.D. (1991). Beyond *Cruzan:* Individual rights, family autonomy and the persistent vegetative state. *Journal of the American Geriatrics Society, 39:* 1018–1024.

Arras, J.D., and Dubler, N.N. (in press, 1995). Ethical and social implications of high-tech home care: An overview. In Arras, J.D. (ed.), *Bringing the Hospital Home: Ethical and Social Implications of High-Tech Home Care.* Baltimore: Johns Hopkins University Press.

Asch, A. (1990). Commentary: Abused or neglected clients—or abusive or neglectful service systems? In R.A. Kane and A.L. Caplan (eds.), *Everyday Ethics: Resolving Dilemmas in Nursing Home Life*, pp. 113–121. New York: Springer Publishing Co.

Blustein, J. (1993). The family in medical decisionmaking. *Hastings Center Report, 23*: 6–13.

Buchanan, A.E., and Brock, D.W. (1989). *Deciding for Others: The Ethics of Surrogate Decision Making*. New York: Cambridge University Press.

Collopy, B.J., Dubler, N.N., and Zuckerman, C. (1990). The ethics of home care: Autonomy and accommodation. *Hastings Center Report, 20* (Special Supplement): 1–16.

Drane, J. (1985). The many faces of competency. *Hastings Center Report, 15*: 17–21.

Dresser, R., and Robertson, J. (1989). Quality of life and treatment decisions for incompetent patients: A critique of the orthodox approach. *Law, Medicine and Health Care, 17*: 234–268.

Dubler, N.N. (1990). Accommodating the home care client: A look at rights and interests. In C. Zuckerman, N.N. Dubler, and B. Collopy (eds.), *Home Health Care Options: A Guide for Older Persons and Concerned Families*, pp. 141–165. New York: Plenum.

Dubler, N.N., and Marcus, L. (1994). *Mediating Bioethical Disputes*. New York: United Hospital Fund of New York.

Hardwig, J. (1990). What about the family? *Hastings Center Report, 20*: 5–10.

Jecker, N. (1993). Impartiality and special relationships. In D.T. Meyer, K. Kipris, and C.F. Murphy (eds.), *Kindred Matters: Rethinking the Philosophy of the Family*, pp. 74–89. Ithaca, N.Y.: Cornell University Press.

Kane, R.A., and Caplan, A.L. (eds.). (1990). *Everyday Ethics: Resolving Dilemmas in Nursing Home Life*. New York: Springer Publishing Co.

Levinsky, N. (1984). The doctor's master. *New England Journal of Medicine, 311*: 1573–1575.

Minow, M. (1990). *Making All the Difference: Inclusion, Exclusion, and American Law*. Ithaca, N.Y.: Cornell University Press.

Moody, H.R. (1992). *Ethics in an Aging Society*. Baltimore: Johns Hopkins University Press.

Nelson, J. (1992). Taking families seriously. *Hastings Center Report, 22*: 6–12.

Nelson, J.L., and Nelson, H.L. (in press, 1994). *The Patient in the Family*, chap. 7. New York: Routledge.

Noddings, N. (in press, 1995). Moral obligation or moral support for high-tech home care. In J.D. Arras (ed.), *Bringing the Hospital Home: Ethical and So-*

cial Implications of High-Tech Home Care. Baltimore: Johns Hopkins University Press.

Veatch, R.M. (1972). Models for ethical medicine in a revolutionary age. *Hastings Center Report, 2:* 5–7.

West, M.B., and Gibson, J.M. (1992). Facilitating medical ethics case review: What ethics committees can learn from mediation and facilitation techniques. *Cambridge Quarterly of Healthcare Ethics, 1:* 63–74.

V PREVENTIVE ETHICS IN LONG-TERM CARE DECISION MAKING

CHAPTER ELEVEN

Managing the Conceptual and Ethical Dimensions
of Long-Term Care Decision Making: A Preventive
Ethics Approach

*Laurence B. McCullough, Nancy L. Wilson, Jill A. Rhymes,
and Thomas A. Teasdale*

This chapter begins where the introductory essay begins, with a useful definition of long-term care as "a set of health, personal care and social services delivered over a sustained period of time to persons who have lost or never acquired some degree of functional capacity" (Kane and Kane, 1987, p. 4). This definition is elegant in its formulation and points, as well, to the complexity of long-term care. The main lesson of the preceding chapters is to underscore—empirically, politically, historically, and therefore ethically—the complexity of decisions about long-term care, that is, about living or support arrangements in response to chronic changes in capacity for self-care. It is clear that this complexity, which is a function of policy constraints, history, medical and social conditions, multiple players and their bonds of obligations straining against self-interest, and other factors discussed in earlier chapters, will defy ready categorization into established theoretical pigeonholes.

Challenging Orthodoxy

Previous chapters have mounted a series of powerful challenges to the adequacy of existing theoretical strategies in the bioethics literature for long-term care decision making. We continue that challenge here, now against the reactive, retrospective approach that analyzes conflicts and proposes solutions for them *after they have occurred*. Ethical conflicts engage us intellectually, but they can and do rend familial relationships and add unnecessary stress to the professional–client/patient relationship. Better for all involved in long-term care decision making that ethical conflicts be prevented. Previous chapters question a wide-ranging set of assumptions about independence and safety, autonomy, familial relationships and obligations, the immunity of our practices and institutions to the influence of history and policy, and decision making about complex, ambiguous matters. This chapter questions the retrospective approach to ethical conflicts that presently dominates the bioethics—and ethics and aging—literature.

We therefore undertake the task of proposing a *preventive ethics strategy* to manage the complexity of the conceptual and ethical dimensions of long-term care decision making in practice, building on the work of our colleagues in the preceding chapters. The implications of the conceptual and ethical dimensions of long-term care are then taken up. We adopt as our point of departure the strategy employed by Bart Collopy (Chap. 7), George Agich (Chap. 6), and John Arras (Chap. 10), namely, to contrast acute-care and long-term care decision making. On this basis we then identify the main conceptual and ethical dimensions of the latter.

The complexity of long-term care decision making need not necessarily disarm those who undertake it: elders, family members, and professionals. They can manage that complexity prospectively, with a view toward preventing ethical conflicts that arise almost as a natural function of the conceptual and ethical dimensions of long-term care decision making. Thus, our main focus in this chapter is on a preventive ethics approach to managing these ambiguities and complexities. This approach is designed to equip the professional working with elders and family members to integrate the conceptual and ethical analyses of the preceding chapters into a practical approach designed to prevent ethical conflict.

Acute versus Long-Term Care

Long-term care differs significantly from acute care. Brian Hofland points out that acute care, as a rule, involves well-defined problems as well as well-defined alternatives for managing them. Long-term care, by contrast, exhibits greater ambiguity. Problems are less well-defined and alternatives therefore more resistant to clear definition (Hofland, 1990). Acute care tends to involve problems that are clear-cut: the patient has poor vascularization secondary to poorly controlled diabetes or occlusion of the coronary arteries. In more technical terms, the patient has or is thought to have an anatomical or physiological abnormality. Pathophysiology falls within the province of the health care professions, medicine in particular. Thus, a built-in feature of acute care is that the health care professional, rather than the patient, possesses the intellectual basis for naming the patient's problem. This dependence on health care professionals to name our problems when we are patients in acute-care settings is one of the sources of the power of health care professionals over patients. This aspect of the healer's power is usually not shared with the patient (Brody, 1992).

The health care professional exercises power in an institutional context in which resources for the diagnosis and management of acute-care problems are organized and made available for health care professionals to use in the care of patients. Health care professionals, not patients, control access to these resources, another source of the physician's power in the acute-care setting.

The health care professional also exercises power within a hierarchical structure, in which, for example, the physician writes orders that other professionals or technologists then carry out. Physicians recommend management strategies to patients. It is no longer the case, however, that physicians or any other health care professionals issue orders to patients, with which compliance is to be "prompt and implicit," as was expected in nineteenth-century American medical ethics (American Medical Association, 1847).

One important implication of the health care professional's role in the acute-care setting, especially in the hospital setting, is that patients experience dependence on their professional caregivers—physicians, nurses, and allied health professionals. This kind of dependence results in a loss of power by the patient. The informed consent process can be understood as a response to enhance the patient's autonomy and therefore presumably the patient's power (McCullough and Wear, 1985).

In summary, in the acute-care setting, the health care professional, the physician in particular, possesses the power to name the patient's problem. The physician thus plays the role of chief ontologist,[1] undertaking diagnostic workups to place the patient's reality into the correct pathophysiological category. The patient cannot perform this role, because the patient lacks the relevant knowledge. Increasingly, third party payers and managers, in addition to the informed consent process, function as significant counterweights to the physician's power.

The patient's pathophysiology and the response of physicians and health care professionals and institutions to it have significant implications for the patient in other spheres of his or her life and for others in the patient's life. However, these are treated as implications—not matters of central concern—of acute care for third parties to the physician-patient relationship. The interests of the patient are therefore separable from those of family members in the acute-care settings. Separable interests raise the problem of conflict of interest discussed earlier by Arras (Chap. 10). Long-term care differs sharply in at least three respects: (*a*) competing realities rather than clearly defined problems; (*b*) less professional control of resources; and (*c*) family interests as intimately intertwined with and not easily separated from those of the elder.

Competing Realities

First, the elder may not be a patient at all. He or she is usually living in some community setting, getting along more or less well enough with his or her life. The physical, mental, or social changes that occur may not be acknowledged by the elder or, if acknowledged, may not be seen as problems by the elder. Yet, family members or the physician may judge these changes to be problems. In short, there is no chief ontologist in long-term care decision making.

For example, older people living alone may regard themselves as quite capable of taking care of themselves, yet their case manager may notice that their nutritional status seems to be deteriorating. The case manager is expected to notice such changes and respond to them as potential threats to the elders' well-being. The elders may resist such solicitous intervention because they do not agree with the case manager's description of their condition or with the case manager's moral judgment that this condition poses a potential risk and therefore ought to be addressed. *Competing realities* constitute a defining feature of long-term care decision making and constitute a major source of ethical conflict within that process, a taxonomy of which was provided by Terrie Wetle (Chap. 4).

The realities of long-term care, as the above example illustrates, have both a factual and an evaluative dimension. The fact that the elders are or might be malnourished or at risk for malnourishment can be in dispute between them and their case manager. What each of them thinks about the importance or urgency of such factual matters can also be in dispute. By training and professional judgment, formed in beneficence-based[2] regard for the well-being of a client, the case manager reaches the evaluation that risk of malnourishment is a harm to these elders and should be prevented. Such judgments possess the power to create dependencies like those created in acute care by the power to name the patient's problem. Yet, in the sort of analysis that Collopy (Chap. 7) offered, the elders' decisions about how they live may be an expression of their own concept of safety. Adequate nourishment, in Agich's (Chap. 6) language, involves the interstitial exercise of autonomy, the cumulative effect of which may be a nodal decision, for example, whether to stay in one's own home or move to a more structured setting in which nourishment is assured.

Thus, the competing realities of long-term care decision making embrace both factual and moral elements, raising two questions: (1) Is there an authoritative factual description of the elder's situation? and (2) What ought the elder, family members, and professionals think of that situation? To the extent that matters of health are at stake, the professional's descriptions in response to the first question possess considerable intellectual authority. The burden of proof would be on the individuals with clinical symptoms of malnourishment to show that they were not, in fact, malnourished. However, there is no smooth transition from intellectually authoritative clinical descriptions in response to the first question above to controlling answers to the second question.

This second question calls for an evaluative judgment about agreed-upon facts; agreement on facts does not by itself produce an agreed-upon evaluative judgment. Evaluative judgments are formed on the basis of different perspectives on the elders' interests. Professionals take a perspective external to that of the elders, i.e., a beneficence-based judgment about what would be good for *any* individual at risk for malnourishment. The elders, exercising autonomy, take their own, internal perspective on these matters. This perspective can be usefully informed—but ought not be controlled—by the professional's perspective.

Professionals, including case managers, therefore need to be aware of their power to control the process that leads to the definition of elders' problems (Wetle, Chap. 4). The preventive ethics strategy that we propose later in this chapter should be read as an antidote to this dimension of the professional's power.

Family members also have a perspective on the elders' interests. In long-term care decision making, as Arras (Chap. 10) argued, family members are not third parties to the decision-making process, especially family members who have been or might become caregivers. Family members are bound to the elder in complex moral relationships, whether as spouses (Jecker, Chap. 8) or children (Brakman, Chap. 9) or in-laws and stepchildren, or other kinship relationships. Family members bound to the elder by ties of moral obligation, which ought to be equal with respect to gender but in practice may not be, are thus the elder's moral intimates. Their perspective is at once external (they see things from a perspective other than that of the elder) and intimate; to the extent that they know the elder well, spouses especially, they have access to the elder's internal perspective on the elder's interests. As Arras (Chap. 10) pointed out, conflict of interest is not a terribly useful conceptualization of this complex moral relationship. Nonetheless, there is surely the potential for confusion of family members' interests, which might be antithetical to those of the elder, in family members' perspectives on the elder's interests.

In the language of philosophical ethics, long-term care decisions involve a kind of moral realism: situations are defined at their core not only from factually informed perspectives but also by the nexus of moral obligations that define the identity of elders and family members and shape the history of their relationships. Moral realism flourished in the eighteenth century in Great Britain (Price, 1948) and took the view that "is" did indeed imply "ought" when the "is" described a social role that was comprised of a nexus of obligations. Moral realism, long out of favor in twentieth-century Anglo-American philosophy, has recently enjoyed something of a renaissance in which moral realities are thought to "supervene" factual realities (Miller, 1992). The older version of moral realism is the more appropriate conceptualization of long-term care decision making: moral realities help to *constitute*—not supervene or somehow add something to—the situations that trigger long-term care decision making.

In acute-care decision making, we saw that there is often a chief ontologist, whose descriptions of the patient's condition possess intellectual authority and whose moral judgments about how that condition ought to be managed can be and are contested by patients. In long-term care decision making both factual and moral elements can be and are contested, a problem to which a preventive ethics approach to long-term care decision making must respond.

Control of Resources

Second, the resources that might be marshaled in response to a situation that is agreed to be a problem are not under the sole control of the health care professional. Most of the resources consumed in long-term care in the United States belong to the so-called informal caregivers, the elder's moral intimates: spouses, children, other kinfolk, stepchildren, in-

laws, neighbors, and friends. These individuals do not live in hierarchical relationships to the elder, nor the elder to them. As Nancy Jecker
(Chap. 8) and Sarah Brakman (Chap. 9) pointed out earlier, the relationships between elders and family members involve tangled, often in-
choate, and negotiable webs of obligations and their limits. Moreover,
the informal caregivers do not stand in hierarchical relationships to professionals or to institutions that arrange or deliver formal long-term care
services. In short, the professional cannot issue orders to family members and other informal caregivers nor they to each other.

Decisions about the use of resources thus lack the drama that often
accompanies such decisions in the acute-care setting, for example,
whether to admit a gravely ill patient with a poor prognosis to an already overused critical care unit. Power is more diffuse and the exercise
of autonomy by elders and family members more subtle and quotidian.
In Agich's (Chap. 6) terms, once nodal decisions have been made, for instance, to stay at home and accept Meals on Wheels to help prevent malnourishment, many matters of interstitial decision making move to the
fore. Harry R. Moody has argued that requests, compromise, and negotiation should be the tools of decision making in long-term care (Moody,
1992). Agich's (Chap. 6) analysis helps us see why: interstitial decision
making among moral intimates, especially when the burden of care is
unequal between genders, involves the subtle skills of negotiation rather
than the blunt exercise of power to resolve nodal questions.

Martha Holstein and Thomas Cole (Chap. 2) and Nancy Wilson
(Chap. 3) demonstrated earlier in this volume that powerful historical
and policy forces affect the nature and availability of resources for long-
term care decision making. History and policy making define, indeed
create, and control access to long-term care resources. That most such
care is provided by family and community members is no accident. Historical stigmas of poverty are associated with nursing homes, and the
lack of publicly funded alternatives de facto exploits the obligations of
spouses, children, kinfolk, and friends. In order to control access to resources, professionals have been empowered to play the role of gatekeepers. Case managers play this role explicitly, as do others, physicians
especially. Rosalie Kane (Chap. 5) and Wetle (Chap. 4) demonstrated
that case managers are increasingly aware of the ethical conflicts gener-
ated by their role as gatekeepers.

Constraints thus do not operate in the background of long-term care
decision making; they define the very parameters of what is realistically

available to elders with long-term care needs. Managing the effect of resource constraints on both nodal and interstitial autonomy of elders and family members and on the constant negotiation and renegotiation of limited obligations to provide care is an essential element of preventive ethics in long-term care decision making.

The Importance of the Psychosocial

Third, the psychosocial spheres of elders' lives cannot be ignored in long-term care decision making, because this process shapes the elders' and family members psychosocial reality. This is because elders' problems, while they may involve mental or physical change, just as often involve social change. Loss of self-sufficiency is frequently a social phenomenon in the life of elders and their moral intimates, not a medical one. Relocating to receive care or accepting assistance with daily tasks may have a profound effect on elders' self-identity and opportunity to perform cherished social roles. Acute care pertains mainly to health matters, while long-term care pertains to health and to housing, income, self-care, community, family, and personal matters (Kane, Chap. 5; Wilson, Chap. 3).

In other words, long-term care decisions are prompted by changes that can pose a direct threat to the self-identity of elders and therefore of family members, spouses especially (Jecker, Chap. 8). In philosophical accounts, self-identity is appropriately addressed in terms of the necessary conditions for the unity of personal identity over time. Such philosophical analysis focuses on whether continuity of physical or mental identity over time is required for self-identity as its necessary condition. These austere philosophical investigations enjoy the luxury of ignoring the material, sufficient conditions for mundane self-identity and are animated by Enlightenment ideals of the unity of persons.

Mundane, quotidian self-identity in its material sense involves long-standing patterns of behavior, expectations, and relationships (including moral obligations as a spouse, parent, or child) (Agich, Chap. 6; Collopy, Chap. 7). Self-identity in its material sense is best understood as a coping strategy with the conditions of human existence at the end of the most violent and rending century in the recorded history of our species. Elders have lived through most of that century, their children a goodly part of it. Self-identity in its material sense aims at social, moral, and aesthetic coherence of who one is and hopes still to be in a sometimes hostile and confusing world. In the language of Irwin Lieb (1991), we can say that self-identity seeks to weave the self-as-past together with the self-as-future well enough, that is, in an effort to avoid destructive tension between the two.

Long-term care decision making sometimes confronts the possibility of such tension. A recent qualitative study of elders' values in long-term care decision making indicates that preservation of self-identify is an important consideration (McCullough et al., 1993). Respondents in this study expressed their values in this category in straightforward terms, e.g., staying in one's own home, not leaving one's neighborhood of many years, etc. These values are often threatened in long-term care decision making.

The decision-making process has more at stake than simply a living setting or care arrangement, because the latter are structured by history, policy, professionals, and institutions in ways not always compatible with maintaining or adapting individual identity. Living independently is a struggle in a nursing home and living securely can be a struggle when living alone in a high-crime area. Whether the elder and family members ought to be willing to embrace long-term care alternatives is thus partly a function of whether they ought to be willing to embrace the psychosocial realities entailed by those alternatives.

Kane (Chap. 5) and Wetle (Chap. 4) identified and examined value-based conflicts in long-term care decision making, the awareness of case managers of those conflicts, and the possibilities of effectively addressing those conflicts in practice. The challenge to the professional who seeks to manage the psychosocial dimensions of long-term care decision making effectively is to practice nondirective counseling about value-laden decisions. The ethos of nondirective counseling has been developed to prevent professionals from imposing their own values on clients and patients, a positive development in the ethics of health care professionals. A dangerous implication of nondirective counseling is to conclude that the professional has no role to play whenever value-laden, normative matters (what ought to be done) are at stake. These, it is thought, are matters for patients and clients to decide on their own. This view of nondirective counseling could amount to a kind of abandonment, especially in the context of long-term care where elders and family members may not have acknowledged that their problems involve competing realities, justified constraints on their own resources, interests, and obligations, and the negotiation of their own self-identity. Nondirective counseling—a key element of preventive ethics strategies—can identify these issues in the constructive and open-ended way called for by long-term care decision making.

Summary

In summary, long-term care decision making involves competing realities, including competing evaluative interpretations of realities. There can be disagreement about whether the mental or physical or social changes that reduce self-sufficiency in ADL have occurred and, when they have occurred, whether they should count as problems. There is no chief ontologist, even when the elder is a patient. The power to name the problem is thus contested, not settled as it is in the acute-care setting. Second, the power to command resources in response to a long-term care problem (once it is agreed to be such) is widely diffused among the elder, informal and formal caregivers, and institutions. Because of the large role that they play, informal caregivers are major long-term care resources and important decision makers with the elder and the physician. The obligations of family members and their legitimate interests and the obligations of elders to family members are essential for deciding whether they ought to serve as such a resource. Third, long-term care is inherently biopsychosocial in nature. Indeed, long-term care decision making, with its competing realities, essentially temporal character, and shifting cast of participants, may best exemplify the biopsychosocial model (Engel, 1980) in health care and social services.

Implications for Practice

Far and away the dominant theme of the previous chapters is ambiguity, including ambiguity introduced by contradiction or the threat of contradiction in the moral lives of elders and those who care for them. These ambiguities shape housing and financial decisions, as well as decisions about what care is needed and who can, will, or ought to provide that care. Long-term care problems and decisions do not lend themselves to abstract clarity; they do not come into a sharp and steady focus. They are blurred, because they are shifting, uncertain, and contested. Any ethical framework for long-term care decision making must therefore make ambiguity the fundamental category and response to ambiguity the appropriate strategy (Arras, 1984).

Ambiguity is not to be resolved or solved. The language of resolution of conflict that figures so prominently in the bioethics literature is therefore inadequate to the ethics of long-term care decision making. Instead, the language of management of ambiguity and its potential to generate conflicting obligations and, therefore, *preventive ethics* moves to the fore.

Manage comes from an Italian root that pertains to the training of horses—the analogue of the ambiguity, conflict, or problem to be managed and prevented. Now, even the most docile and well-trained of horses can turn ornery without warning. The rider does not control a horse as if the rider were in charge. The rider attends to the horse's signals and responds to them, directing the horse, coaxing, on the alert to the unexpected. The relationship between horse and rider is one of ongoing negotiation and prevention of worst outcomes. The same is true for long-term care decision making.

Long-term care decision making thus does not lend itself to the theoretical resolution of establishing *a priori,* that is, without reference to experience, a fixed hierarchy of ethical principles and then applying that hierarchy to cases. Moreover, decision making under conditions of ambiguity is best understood as a fragile process, open to both success and failure, and thus open as well to the need for reactivating the decision-making process when failure occurs. The most appropriate responses of the professional assisting elders and families with long-term care decision making are to be aware of the ambiguities of long-term care decision making and to take a preventive ethics posture toward conflicting obligations and ambiguity.

A preventive ethics approach to long-term care decision making will be described in the next section. The authors of the previous chapters have identified the following conceptual and ethical issues that must be addressed in and by this decision-making process:

1. Powerful system constraints at the macrolevel of policy (Wilson, Chap. 3) are shaped by a long and implacable history (Holstein and Cole, Chap. 2) and, in turn, shape the long-term care decision-making process (Kane, Chap. 5; Wetle, Chap. 4; Wilson, Chap. 3).

2. There are also constraints operating at the microlevel of the decision-making process. These include such factors as a shifting cast of decision makers, decision making as a hurried process depending on the urgency of the elder's need or the family's limits, and failure sometimes to appreciate that a decision needs to be made (Kane, Chap. 5).

3. These two factors combine with the powerful element of gender bias, leading to the provision of long-term care as a way of life for some women (Jecker, Chap. 8; Wilson, Chap. 3).

4. Constraints on the professional's role include competing realities, time, uncertainty about who is the primary client, the preferences of elders and family members, and multiple roles and "agencies" played by the professional (Wetle, Chap. 4).

5. All of the constraints on long-term care decision making can impair the exercise of autonomy, both nodal and interstitial (Agich, Chap. 6). However, even implacable constraints on nodal autonomy do not entail such constraints on interstitial autonomy (Agich, Chap. 6). This represents a significant opportunity to enhance autonomy both of elder and family.

6. There are competing realities, which should be understood as a complex mix of both factual and moral matters. The latter include the following:

   a. Concern for safety seems to override all other considerations or values (Kane, Chap. 5), reflecting—and potentially reinforced by— the dominance of beneficence-based judgments of professionals (Wetle, Chap. 4).

   b. Safety should not be seen as an independent value but on a continuum with the autonomy-based value of independence (Collopy, Chap. 7).

7. In contrast to the acute-care model, family members may be full participants in both caregiving and decision making and have legitimate, even if conflicting, interests of their own and should not be considered third parties disabled by conflicts of interest (Arras, Chap. 10).

8. The obligations of spouses (Jecker, Chap. 8) and adult children (Brakman, Chap. 9)—indeed, of any long-term caregiver—are limited.

9. Elders, therefore, have obligations to family members and other caregivers to respect their legitimate interests (Arras, Chap. 10).

10. The complex nexus of obligations and interests joining the parties to long-term care decision making cannot be settled *a priori,* that is, in theory. This complexity and its moral ambiguities must be negotiated for each case and may result in a trial of a long-term care arrangement as the outcome.

11. Long-term care decision making is a fragile process, subject to periodic breakdowns and the consequent need to restart the decision-making process (Kane, Chap. 5).

12. The professional can play the crucial role of initiating, in a nondirective fashion, consideration of the ethical dimensions of long-term care decision making, a practice implication of *all* of the preceding chapters.

A Preventive Ethics Approach to Long-Term Care Decision Making

Preventive ethics (Chervenak and McCullough, 1990; Forrow, Arnold, and Parker, 1993) eschews theoretical, *a priori* resolutions of the ambiguous and complex process of long-term care decision making. Preventive ethics takes a prospective approach to ethical conflict in the decision-making process. The preceding analysis of the conceptual and ethical dimensions of long-term care decision making and their implications for practice makes it possible to describe a preventive ethics approach to long-term care decision making. This preventive ethics approach individualizes decision making, thus creating a powerful antidote to the "cookie cutter" care plans against which Kane (Chap. 5) cautioned earlier in this volume.

This approach is designed to check the potentially overriding power of beneficence-based professional judgment, especially about safety of the elder, and to maximize respect for the legitimate interests, limited obligations, and autonomy of elders and family members. Any particular long-term care arrangement that results from this decision-making process will be open to review and renegotiation.

By the time the professional becomes involved in the process, some long-term care decisions, nodal as well as interstitial, have already been made, seriously considered, or firmly rejected. Professional involvement in the long-term care decision-making process can sometimes unintentionally fracture relationships and "careers" of caring. Using the following preventive ethics approach, the professional can, in a nondirective fashion, bring some structure and order to both nodal and interstitial long-term care decisions. While the elements of this preventive ethics approach are listed in a particular order, the process itself may not always be linear.

1. Identify the stakeholders in the decision. Who should be included in the process?

2. Seek an *agreed-upon factual account* of the elder's condition, especially significant or irreversible changes in capacity for self-care.

a. Identify the biopsychosocial needs and care requirements of the elder.

b. Identify whether family members are physically and cognitively able to meet those requirements.

3. Identify *formal long-term care services that are realistically available* to meet the elder's needs, given financial, geographic, and policy constraints.

a. Identify the benefits of and risks of each alternative, to prevent making the assumption that an alternative (especially the nursing home) is risk-free.

4. Invite elder and family members, on the basis of their evaluations, to identify *all reasonable alternatives.*

a. Invite discussion of reasonable, justified limits of familial obligations to provide care to elder.

b. Invite recognition of gender bias in the family's distribution of caregiving burden and expectations of who can and ought to provide long-term care.

c. Elicit elder's views about obligation to prevent unreasonable caregiving burdens on family members, especially female family members.

5. Elicit the *values of the elder and family members,* and on this basis elicit their *evaluations* of the elder's condition and realistic alternatives for its management.

a. Remind elder and family members that there is usually more than one alternative consistent with their values.

b. Encourage elder and family members to identify and take account of each other's limited obligations to protect and promote the interests of others, as an important basis for evaluating realistic alternatives.

c. Invite careful and thoughtful discussion of the implications of realistic alternatives for self-identity of elder and family members, especially for relationships that they want to protect and promote.

6. If the professional has recommendations—either from among these alternatives or for one that has been set aside—the professional should *offer recommendations.*

a. When possible, recommendations should be based primarily on what appears to be in the elder's and family members' interests, rather than on agency or institutional interests.

7. Encourage *agreement on an alternative, recognizing that it may not be permanent.*

 a. Remind elder and family members that the long-term care arrangement selected may not work.

 b. Encourage elder and family members to establish a process for review of the arrangement and, if possible, the criteria for its stopping/continuation/revision.

This preventive ethics approach to long-term care decision making takes seriously the time constraints that can affect the decision-making process. One result of time constraints is that some decisions may already have been made. But these should not be regarded as irrevocable, and the elder and family member could be asked if they want to review or reconsider the decision already made. In addition, they should be made aware that even when nodal decisions of long-term care have been made, many everyday or interstitial decisions remain to be made, and these decisions can be made in a way that takes account of the elder's and family members' interests. That some nodal decisions may have, in effect, been made for the elder or family does not require that subsequent everyday decisions be made for them.

The above decision-making process should be attempted for elders with diminished decision making capacity, as a way to determine if they can make their own decisions. The kinds of skills called for in the above process are not necessarily well measured by existing, validated mental status assessment instruments. If elders or family members show themselves irreversibly unable to participate in the above decision-making process, then that process should be initiated with others acting as proxies for the elders or family members. The proxy should be asked to focus primarily on the elder's or family member's values and preferences, as best as these can be known. There will be some distance between the actual autonomy of the elder or family member and any surrogate, but this distance is not totally insurmountable. Conscientious proxy decision making should be the goal, not perfect proxy decision making; the latter is simply an impossible standard to which to hold anyone.

We find the reservations of Arras (Chap. 10) about a "low-key, oblique approach" to long-term care decision making persuasive. Thus, the preventive ethics approach described above takes an open approach to that process. This approach to long-term care decision making should, like any clinical intervention, be offered to elders and family members and their consent elicited to undertake the process.

Implications of Preventive Ethics for Policy and Planning

The preventive ethics approach to long-term care decision making that we have proposed here has important, still fully to be identified and explored implications for public policy and for institutional practice and planning. Public policy and institutional practice and policies can sometimes function synergistically as a source of unnecessary and ethically suspect impediments to preventive ethics. When they do so they should be challenged and forced to bear the burden of proof of the ethical justification for the exercise of such considerable power. In short, rethinking the conceptual and ethical dimensions of microlevel long-term care decision making will, as it progresses, create a policy and practice agenda of reform of macrolevel long-term care decision making.

Implications for Bioethics: Challenges from the Periphery to the Core

Laurence McCullough and Nancy Wilson noted in Chapter 1 that, until very recently, the literature on ethics and aging has been dominated by end-of-life decision making. They invited the reader to consider the subsequent chapters to be a corrective to this distortion of the ethics of aging and a complement to the growing literature on ethics in long-term care decision making. We believe that these chapters have delivered on this promise. They have also accomplished much more: they have charted the conceptual and ethical dimensions of long-term care decision making in a way that takes seriously and builds on empirical studies, as well as on the lessons of history and policy.

Long-term care decision making by elders, family members, and professionals calls for more than routine responses, because the changes that prompt long-term care decisions dislodge elders and family from the nexus of relationships, achievements, sacrifices, and other factors from and in which human beings sustain their identities and worlds of meaning. A spouse dies or a child reaches the limits of caregiving obligations and support networks unravel. Previously accommodated levels of dependence can no longer be accommodated. The elder confronts a world in which self-identity must be adapted to increased levels of dependence. The adult children confront a world in which endless sacrifice may shape or shatter their self-identity. An elder, for example, hospitalized with pneumonia experiences worsening of her congestive heart failure and mental status changes. The discharge planner suggests to the patient's daughter that her mother will need a significant level of support and supervision if she is to return to her ranch in the hill country, hours away from the city where her daughter lives and works. The issues go beyond where and how to live. The issues become the challenge to this woman and her daughter to forge a caregiving relationship that will shape the self-identity of both.

In short, long-term care decisions reach into the nooks and crannies of the moral lives of elders and their families, because self-identity permeates our moral lives. The moral life, as philosophers since Socrates have taught, comprises our obligations to others, because acknowledging and fulfilling obligations shape each individual's identity. Forging, and through negotiation reforging, caregiver obligations and care receiver obligations shape and reshape self-identity, that is, one's moral life. Long-term care decision making thus roils with complexity, ambiguity, conflict, and stress, just as the moral life generally roils with complexity, ambiguity, conflict, and stress.

Complexity, ambiguity, conflict, and stress are, to put it simply, the normal conditions of the moral life. These features of our moral lives cannot be "solved," that is, eliminated. They are, instead, to be managed—we cope with and adapt to them as best we can, by shaping a self-identity in which one still can recognize oneself and intimate others. And so elders and family members often dedicate themselves to the moral work of long-term care decision making.

This work and the help professionals and institutions offer go on at the periphery of acute, high-tech health care, not at its core. Traditional bioethics has been largely a creature of acute, high-tech medical care. Thus, it is no surprise that long-term care decision making is at the periphery, not the core, of traditional bioethics.

At the core of bioethics, as at the core of acute, high-tech medicine, things are conceptually crisp and tidy. Patients all have diagnostic labels, and interventions are applied routinely in response to diagnoses. Power and authority, similarly, are crisp and tidy; physicians and, increasingly, hospitals and managed care companies originate power and share it with patients, but physicians remain in authority. Patients are, at most, an authority. Families, already at risk for conflicts of interest, are also at risk for loss of power and authority. Complexity, ambiguity, conflict, and stress are not defining features of acute care; they are problems to be managed to a minimum and, ideally, eliminated. Traditional bioethics, the ready servant of acute, high-tech medicine, has largely—and uncritically—bought into this understanding of acute care, reinforcing it with the insistence on philosophical crispness and tidiness.

The commitment to conceptual crispness and tidiness at the core of bioethics reinforces the abstractness of acute, high-tech medicine (McCullough, 1989). Acute, high-tech medicine conceptualizes patients under categories of disease and their natural histories. The individuality of patients counts little in clinical judgment, despite the rhetoric of medicine to the contrary (McCullough, 1991). Acute, high-tech bioethics conceptualizes patients under ethical principles such as autonomy and self-determination. But these are the same in all of us and do not mark us out as individuals. Both acute, high-tech medicine and its bioethics ignore the relationship of patients to others, relationships that help to establish self-identity. Increasingly, patients are conceptualized as strangers, disconnected from health care professionals and from family and community (Engelhardt, 1986; Rothman, 1990).

In contrast, at the periphery of acute care and its bioethics, in long-term care decision making we find concrete, actual elders and family members doing the work of the moral life in response to far-reaching, serious challenges. Professionals represent and hold the power to control formal long-term care services, a power that introduces the constraints of history and policy into the everyday lives of elders and family members. The concreteness of this work is implacable, and the preceding chapters embrace that concreteness, attempting to understand it.

The effect of this concreteness is that the periphery of bioethics challenges its core. Patients and their families are not abstractions. Their moral lives come with them to the tertiary surgical and intensive care centers that modern hospitals have become. Their moral lives are challenged by what physicians, nurses, and allied health professionals say and do in these great centers of knowledge and skill. The changes in health status that patients bring to the hospital do not occupy the periphery of patients' lives. Those events are not, in Aristotle's language, accidental determinations of being. They are essential determinations of individual self-identity.

A physician tells a patient he has end-stage heart disease. His heart is failing, and only a transplant gives him a chance to survive, the physician explains, just as the canons of informed consent require her to do. The patient confronts his death and the "harvesting" of someone else's heart to be put in his chest. A physician tells a pregnant woman that to-colysis has failed to prevent premature labor at twenty-five weeks gestational age, that her fetus is in severe distress, and that a cesarean delivery is indicated. She consents and enters the months-long vigil in the neonatal intensive care unit. Her central nervous system–injured child "graduates" from the neonatal intensive care unit into a long-term care relationship with her and her husband. The crisp and tidy self-description of acute, high-tech medicine and of bioethical "issues" is an invitation to self-deception.

The antidote from the periphery is the following. Complexity, ambiguity, conflict, and stress become fundamental conceptual tools. The move to abstractness is supplanted by an insistence on concreteness. The stakes for health care and a bioethics adequate to it become clear: the moral lives of patients, their families, health care professionals, and health care institutions and how those moral lives are shaped and re-shaped in our turbulent world.

NOTES

1. Ontology is the philosophical study of basic categories of reality.

2. Beneficence is an ethical principle that directs the health care professional to seek the greater balance of goods over harms for the patients, as those goods and harms are understood from a rigorous clinical perspective. Beneficence thus takes a perspective that is external to the individual perspective that an individual patient takes on his or her interests. This internal perspective is captured by the ethical principle of respect for autonomy (Beauchamp and McCullough, 1984).

REFERENCES

American Medical Association. (1847). Code of medical ethics. *Transactions of the National Medical Convention 1846–1847*: 83–106.

Arras, J. (1984). Toward an ethic of ambiguity. *Hastings Center Report, 14*: 25–33.

Beauchamp, T.L., and McCullough, L.B. (1984). *Medical Ethics: The Moral Responsibilities of Physicians*. Englewood Cliffs, N.J.: Prentice-Hall.

Brody, H. (1992). *The Healer's Power*. New Haven, Conn.: Yale University Press.

Chervenak, F.A., and McCullough, L.B. (1990). Clinical guides to preventing ethical conflicts between pregnant women and their physicians. *American Journal of Obstetrics and Gynecology, 162*: 303–307.

Engel, G. (1980). The clinical application of biopsychosocial models. *American Journal of Psychiatry, 137*(5): 535–544.

Engelhardt, H.T., Jr. (1986). *The Foundations of Bioethics.* New York: Oxford University Press.

Forrow, L., Arnold, R.M., and Parker, L.S. (1993). Preventive ethics: Expanding the horizons of clinical ethics. *Journal of Clinical Ethics,* 4: 287–294.

Hofland, B. (1990). Introduction. *Generations, 14*(Supplement), 5–8.

Kane, R.A., and Kane, R.L. (1987). *Long-Term Care: Principles, Programs, and Policies.* New York: Springer Publishing Co.

Lieb, I.C. (1991). *Past, Present, and Future: A Philosophical Essay about Time.* Urbana: University of Illinois Press.

McCullough, L.B. (1989). The abstract character and transforming power of medical language. *Soundings, 72:* 111–125.

McCullough, L.B. (1991). Particularism in medicine. *Criticism, 32:* 361–370.

McCullough, L.B., and Wear, S. (1985). Respect for autonomy and medical paternalism reconsidered. *Theoretical Medicine, 6:* 295–308.

McCullough, L.B., Wilson, N.L., Teasdale, T.A., Kolpakchi, A.L., and Skelly, J.R. (1993). Mapping personal, familial, and professional values in long-term care decisions. *Gerontologist, 33:* 324–332.

Miller, R.W. (1992). Moral realism. In L.C. Becker and C.B. Becker (eds.), *Encyclopedia of Ethics,* pp. 847–852. New York: Garland Publishing Co.

Moody, H.R. (1992). *Ethics in an Aging Society.* Baltimore: Johns Hopkins University Press.

Price, R. (1948). *A Review of the Principal Questions in Morals.* Oxford: Oxford University Press. (Reprint of 1787 3rd edition.)

Rothman, D.J. (1990). *Strangers at the Bedside: A History of How Law and Bioethics Transformed Medical Decision Making.* New York: Basic Books.

Index

Library of Congress Cataloging-in-Publication Data

Long-term care decisions : ethical and conceptual dimensions / edited by Laurence B.
    McCullough and Nancy L. Wilson.
        p.   cm.
    Includes bibliographical references and index.
    ISBN 0-8018-4993-4 (alk. paper : hc)
    1. Aged—Long-term care—Moral and ethical aspects—Congresses.   2. Long-term care
of the sick—Moral and ethical aspects—Congresses.   I. McCullough, Laurence B.
II. Wilson, Nancy L. (Nancy Lee), 1952–   .
    [DNLM: 1. Long-Term Care—in old age—congresses.   2. Ethics, Medical—
congresses.   3. Decision Making—congresses.   WT 30 L8476 1995]
RC954.3.L66   1995
362.1'6'0846—dc20
DNLM/DLC
for Library of Congress   94-37416